£3 -
ged

18|5.

The Complete Book of Good Health

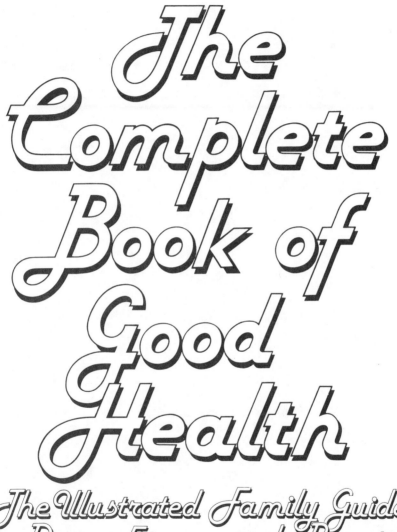

The Complete Book of Good Health

The Illustrated Family Guide to Diet, Fitness and Beauty

Edited by Phoebe Phillips & Pamela Hatch
Introduction by Alexandra Penney

Thomas Y. Crowell, Publishers
Established 1834 New York

This work was first published in Great Britain under the title
THE BEST OF GOOD HEALTH.

THE COMPLETE BOOK OF GOOD HEALTH

Copyright © 1978
by Phoebe Phillips

FIRST U.S. EDITION

ISBN: 0690017812

LIBRARY OF CONGRESS CATALOG CARD NUMBER: 784768

Contributors and Consultants

Contributors
Alexandra Penney, Introduction
Leslie Kenton
Jennie Glew
Dr. Eric Trimmer

Edited by
Phoebe Phillips
Pamela Hatch

Consultants
Dee Remmington
David Prowse
Mary Perigoe
Geoffrey Treissman
Ronald Fread
Dr. Lawrence Wisham
Lorraine Johnson, Designer
Lorna Winslow, Illustrator

Contents

Contents

Contents

Contents

Introduction

A LOOK AT GOOD HEALTH
BY ALEXANDRA PENNEY

Some people think that the last full-scale revolution in this country took place in 1776. They're about 202 years off the mark. The year 1978 marks the moment when the health revolution came into in full swing in the United States. Today, city streets are clogged with joggers. Health clubs are considered as standard built-ins for new apartment housing. Spanking fresh fruit and vegetable stands are popping up on every neighborhood street corner as well as in prime real estate locations. Organic food stores are being built bigger than the biggest supermarkets. And yogurt is crowding out Danish on morning coffee carts.

It started, as everything else seems to have, in the early sixties when young people were questioning just about every facet of the American lifestyle including the national craving for sweets and the sweeping tendency toward paunch. The revolution took real root in the early seventies and today we admit that it is here to stay and making significant changes in the way we live our lives.

The revolution has changed our thinking about our bodies and our minds. Even our language has changed. We were always somewhat aware of calories but now we're conscious of carbohydrates, fats, minerals and trace elements. Protein has become a word as common as candy once was. Cholesterol counts and high bulk or high fiber and low blood sugar are things we definitely ought to know about. Meditation, relaxation

techniques, Sufi and autogenic training may sound somewhat exotic, but to many they're just part of everyday life.

In California it's common to consult weekly with one's nutritionist and to shop in the world's largest health food store, which is open 20 hours a day and takes up a huge three acres of rich Los Angeles loam. Holistic health centers dedicated to the 'whole person' are springing up all over the state. They offer vitamin and herbology courses, psychological insights, naturalistic healing, as well as exercize and massage seminars. Usually these centers are oversubscribed.

In New York the chic-est parties are those to which you wear your leotard, get a tough two hour workout and then relax with some vintage apple juice. You try (as I did), to join the local 'Y' and you are the 803rd woman on the waiting list. All across the country the mood swing is to health and fitness.

Almost daily contact with doctors in all fields has further convinced me of the enormity of the health revolution from coast to coast. The new emphasis on all medical fronts is preventive medicine – instead of waiting until we fall ill, doctors are trying to prevent illness. There are two areas that preventive medicine centers on. The first is a concern with nutrition, eating habits, awareness of foods and their preparation. Special diets for preventive health reasons are just beginning to be central issues at contemporary research centers. 'Nutrition has always been a branch of medicine that has been in slight disrepute. Years ago all the nuts and quacks were in it. Today it is an area of intense interest,' says the chief of a well-known weight control research clinic.

The other area preventive medicine is addressing now is that of physical fitness. For example, if certain stresses can be prevented or at least understood, many medical problems, including heart disease, ulcers, colds, skin problems and much else can be alleviated. The key to solving stress related ailments as well as many other contemporary medical problems may lie in preventing them altogether by emphasizing physical fitness.

It's interesting to note that even today, there is no agreed-upon definition of physical fitness. We are just beginning to investigate what physical fitness is all about and what it can, ultimately, do for each of us. However there is complete agreement that some form of exercise is absolutely essential to physical well-being, and most experts would add that it is essential to mental health as well.

Intimately involved with physical fitness is the relatively new field of sports medicine. Once the province of a handful of doctors who were not taken very seriously, sports medicine is now an area of great significance. If we know how athletes respond to exercise and training, some of this knowledge can be used for the benefit of us all.

Good nutrition and fitness are the twin physical structures underlying good health. But good health has other enormous benefits besides the most obvious ones. *If you're healthy you look good*. If you're eating well, relaxing right and exercising enough, you look trim, attractive and appealing no matter what your age or what features you were born with. It's important to remember, the experts tell us, that you're never too young or never too old to start getting into good shape. Many men and women well above 50 have just begun to exercise in a serious way for the first time in their lives and they can see visible benefits as well as psychological ones.

Another phenomenon of the health revolution is the unprecendented outpouring of books, magazines, articles and medical coverage on the subject. We have reached a point where, for most of us, there is almost too much information to take in. Specialized books on every area of nutrition, exercise, beauty, weight control, fitness and sports are constantly vying for our attention. A journalist who writes frequently on the subject of health has estimated that 'to know everything important on the health scene today would mean at least $2^1/_2$ hours of reading every night and severe eyestrain by day.' *The Complete Book of Good Health* is the answer to that problem. It is a guide to all that one needs to know in general about the state of the art of health today. But, most importantly, it gives enough specialized information to enable one to choose a specific diet, a specific type of exercise, or a particular technique of relaxing with well-founded confidence. *The Complete Book of Good Health* presents, in a concise and understandable manner, every facet of all the areas considered essential to good health today.

WHERE DO WE BEGIN?

For almost all of us, good health was a simple equation learned long ago in school: if you came down with a disease or had an accident, you were in bad health; if not, you were in good health. And that was that! We seemed to float along naturally healthy until struck down by a germ – or a bus – and then a doctor was consulted, to cure us if he could, and console the next of kin if he couldn't.

But, now we know good health – really *good* health – means much more than just not being sick or physically incapacitated. The difference between a 'not sick' person and a truly healthy one is rather like the difference between an oil-and-dirt-clogged old jalopy and a sparkling-clean, smooth-running limousine. Both will probably get you to the supermarket or to church on Sunday morning, but life would be so much more pleasant if you could drive the luxury model.

Today, statistics show that the average man can expect to live to be 73 years old; the average woman, 77. Most of the killer diseases can be cured or at least controlled by modern medicine, and therefore, it is within the power of each one of us to take steps to help the medical world to help us. But more important, it is within the control of each one of us to lead not only 'not sick' lives, but really healthy ones. If we can expect to live more than 70 years, it is virtually imperative to try to attain the best health possible so that we can remain as physically and mentally active as we possibly can be throughout our lives.

This book is designed to teach men, women, and children how to find good health through nutrition, physical fitness, looking their best, and a positive outlook. It is not a medical dictionary with descriptions of symptoms and instructions for cures. It's for those of us who perhaps might be like the clogged old car – not sick, but not working at our best.

Here is an armful of ideas, for every part of your life. There are five parts, each dealing with a major area of Good Health

Part I: **TAKE A GOOD LOOK** prepares you for getting into shape. Charts and graphs have been designed to help you decide how much you should weigh, how you should stand and carry yourself, and, in general, how that intricate machine, your body, works.

Part II: **DIET AND NUTRITION** provides an overall view of how food relates to health. First, it gives a crash course in basic nutrition and includes a number of regimes such as vegetarianism, high bulk, high protein, and natural foods dieting which allow you to eat in a variety of ways yet still with sound nutrition. Special diets are also provided for many food-related problems from the most common (overweight and underweight) to the more obscure like low-blood sugar and the special nutritional problems of teenagers and children. The pros and cons of not eating or fasting are also considered.

Part III: **FAMILY FITNESS** is a detailed discussion of the importance of exercise for overall good health. Regular exercise is a necessity, and included here are a number of ways to easily integrate exercise into your daily life. Discussions of more than forty sports are included with an account of the extent of physical exertion and skill required, clothing and equipment needed, and any special advice or warning a particular sport might warrant.

Nothing is more beautiful than a human being in excellent health. Eating well and keeping your body fit are basics, but a number of extra measures can be taken to give you the best physical presence possible. Part IV: **LOOKING GOOD** gives down-to-earth advice on just that, from literally top to toe. Posture is a sure sign of good health and certainly a significant aspect of good looks, and this section begins with a discussion of this aspect of your overall appearance. It then goes on to discuss the health and beauty care of hair, eyes, ears, skin and feet — both for men and for women.

Finally, good health means more than just the well-being of the body; one's mind and spirit must be functioning as smoothly as one's body. In Part V, **MIND AND BODY TOGETHER**, a number of the more general aspects of everyday life — sex, marriage, family life, living alone, getting older, job and money problems — are talked about in relation to overall health and well-being.

So here is your basic reference guide, to be used frequently by every member of the family. Keep it next to your dictionary and your best loved cookbook; it will be a handy directory to everything you need to make your life not only healthier, but happier.

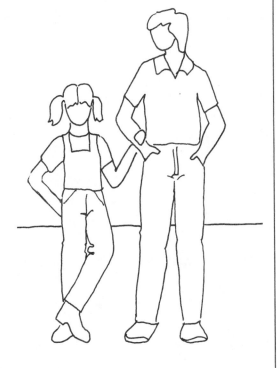

Take
A Good Look

Introduction

GETTING STARTED

We've tried to make it as easy as possible by giving you road maps all along the way, charts and guides to help you plan your trip, enough information to let you decide which route you will take to get there, and signs whenever danger threatens, or conditions require extra caution. The transport is ready, the road ahead is pretty clear, and it's the driver's turn to go through a check list and make sure everything is ready to go.

This section is your check list, or if you prefer, your work sheet. It's all there for you to copy out or fill in the book. We hope you make a separate progress chart for everyone in the family, because that's what family health is all about – not just for women worried about losing weight or looking beautiful, although those are both admirable and helpful goals. It's for husbands, sons, daughters and mothers, aunts and grandparents – in short, everyone you care about, and want to have around feeling good and looking well, enjoying life with renewed energy and vitality for as long as possible.

Copy the charts, on paper large enough to remind you to fill in the spaces every day, every week, or every month.

Pulse rate
You'll see that one of the most important entries asks you to put down your pulse rate, first when resting, then after exercise. We know that your pulse rate is the real key to your heart and lung activity, the cardiovascular condition that will tell you whether or not you are really fit, and keep

tabs on your progress as you get fitter and healthier each month. So learn to take your pulse; sit down comfortably in an armchair, with your arm slightly bent resting on the arm of the chair. Take your opposite hand and put your fingers lightly around your wrist, using your middle fingers to lie just below the base of the thumb. Don't press too hard, but enough to feel the pulse easily.

Most pulse rates are given in beats per minute, so it helps if the hand you are using to take your pulse has a wristwatch, face upwards, with a second hand. Or make sure there's a clock with a second hand within easy view as you sit, without having to crane your neck or stretch your body. It's actually more accurate and easier to keep count for 15 seconds only, and then multiply the answer by four.

The normal pulse rate can vary, but sitting down quietly it should be anywhere from around 71 to 80. Do check with your doctor if it is very different, because you may not realize that your rate has always been high or low, and there is no point in worrying unnecessarily!

After you have taken your pulse resting quietly, run fairly briskly but not too fast up a flight of stairs and down again. That should be your minute of mild exercise; then sit down and take your pulse again immediately. Immediately is the word – let it go for even half a minute, and it will start to drop again.

For 10 minutes of harder exercise, run in place, or do the step text, stepping up with one foot after another on to the bottom step of a staircase and down again. You can use a heavy book or two instead, but make sure you can stand steadily without falling over. Take your pulse immediately as soon as the ten minutes are up.

The fitter you are, the lower your normal pulse rate will be, and the less it will go up after exercise. After the one minute test, your pulse shouldn't rise above 90 beats a minute, or 23 in 15 seconds. Even after ten minutes hard work, it shouldn't be more than 160. You will see a drop in your pulse rate every few pounds you lose, and every day you exercise your body and get things working right. Gradually as you become fitter, even your ordinary pulse rate will drop.

Your weight matters, too, and not just for looks. Every pound adds extra bulk to your fat deposits, and makes it that much harder for your circulation to work properly, for your heart to pump blood, for your muscles to become lithe and smooth. But do keep a sense of proportion; you'll see from the weight check that the shaded areas are all normal limits for that particular age group and height. Use your common sense — if you are pleased with the way you look, if you feel well, and the pulse rate test shows you're fit, then don't agonize if you're on the shady border. Just make sure it doesn't creep up into fatland.

The remaining assessment pointers are there to show you some of the areas where fitness matters most. Your overall condition is vital, so is your attention to skin and hair health. Feet matter — we tell you all about that later

— and so does your feeling of vitality and contentment. Everyone is a complicated system, interconnected and linked up like an electricity grid system. As you see where the problems are and start to do something about them, everything else will improve, too.

A monthly progress chart is an amazingly useful guide to make every week count. Giving yourself impossible goals will never work — you'll only get discouraged, and give up the whole thing. Set yourself a target you think you can reach. Not too easy, mind you, or you won't bother to try, but not so hard you'll get discouraged. If it's calories you're using, put the numbers down, if it's carbohydrates you're counting, put *that* down. Check your daily intake every week, and make sure you haven't strayed off the straight and narrow, forgetting to exercise, letting the meals get over-rich. This is your watchdog. Keep him happy.

Finally, a year planner, a unique and special gift to help you see every month ahead, and plan your fitness goal like a campaign. Use it as a normal diary, too — pin it up on the wall and start whenever you want to. But use it regularly — it's there to remind you of where you can go, now that you've taken a *very* good look …

Assessment Check Asse.

CHECKPOINTS					
NORMAL RANGE	M	F	M	F	M
HEART & LUNGS					
Pulse rate when resting	$^{80}/_{85}$ Variable	$^{85}/_{90}$	$^{85}/_{90}$ Variable	$^{85}/_{90}$	$^{75}/_{75}$
Pulse rate after 1 min mild exercise	100	110	100	110	95
Pulse rate after 10 min hard exercise	$^{130}/_{140}$	$^{130}/_{140}$	130	130	130
Blood pressure; Systolic Diostolic	$^{100}/_{65}$		$^{105}/_{70}$		$^{110}/_{70}$
WEIGHT (See p26-27)					

CONDITION – THE LINE INDICATES NORMAL PROGRESSION WITH AGE

MUSCLES & JOINTS
- Very supple
- Sometimes a little stiff
- Very stiff
- Seldom aching
- Often aching

SKIN & FLESH
- Sometimes spotty
- Often spotty
- Smooth, elastic firm
- Some lines & wrinkles
- Very wrinkled

FEET
- Trim ankles, never swollen unless injured

  Pr

- Often swollen aching, painful

HAIR & NAILS
- Smooth, glossy

- Thinning, fragile

	26-37		38-50		51-65		66-	
F	M	F	M	F	M	F	M	F
75/80	70/75 70-80	70/80	75/80 75-85	75/85	75/85 75-85	75/85	75/85 75-85	75/85
100	95	100	110	110	110	110	110	110
130	130	130	130	130	130	130	130	130
20/70	120/70	130/70	130/80	145/85	155/90	165/90	170/95	

man

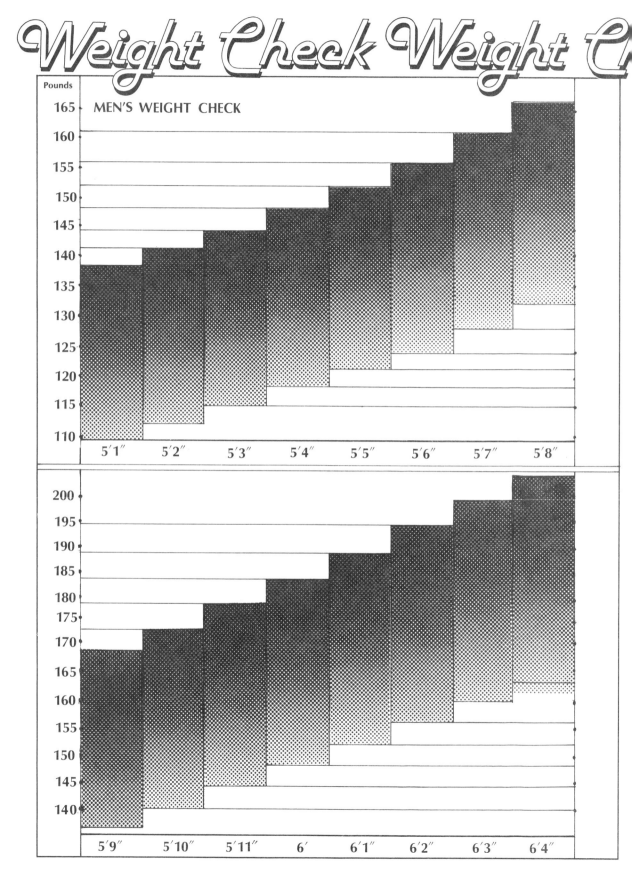

Pounds

MEN'S WEIGHT CHECK

165
160
155
150
145
140
135
130
125
120
115
110

5'1" 5'2" 5'3" 5'4" 5'5" 5'6" 5'7" 5'8"

200
195
190
185
180
175
170
165
160
155
150
145
140

5'9" 5'10" 5'11" 6' 6'1" 6'2" 6'3" 6'4"

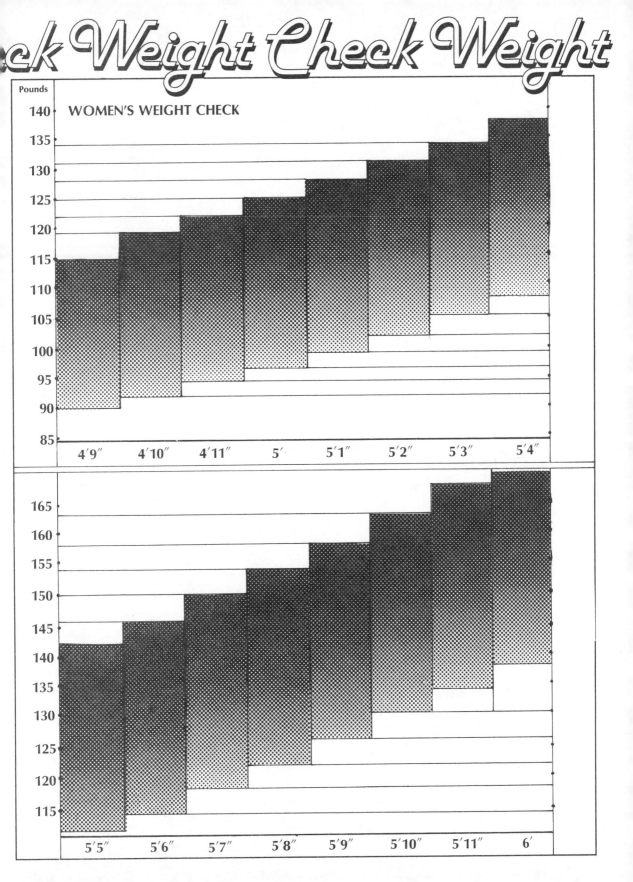

Pounds

WOMEN'S WEIGHT CHECK

140
135
130
125
120
115
110
105
100
95
90
85

4'9" 4'10" 4'11" 5' 5'1" 5'2" 5'3" 5'4"

165
160
155
150
145
140
135
130
125
120
115

5'5" 5'6" 5'7" 5'8" 5'9" 5'10" 5'11" 6'

Progress Check Progres

This is your personal check chart, to keep you going towards the goal of fitness and health. It will help you to see exactly where you are now, and where you want to be in a year. And while you are getting there, it will give you a month-by-month count-down to encourage you every step of the way. Copy the basic chart onto a piece of paper big enough to catch your eye every time you're tempted to eat another piece of cake or forget about that brisk walk you need so much. You'll need a new chart every month, and one for every member of the family who is trying for a better, more exciting and healthier life.

First fill in the column under *now*; be honest! Check blood pressure with your doctor; once a month should be enough, unless you have a problem.

	NOW	FIRST WEEK	
WEIGHT			
HEART & LUNGS Pulse rate resting Pulse rate 1 min after exertion Pulse rate 10 min after exertion Breathless seldom? Often? Never? Blood pressure too high? Too low? Normal?			
RELAXATION & ENERGY Fall asleep easily, wake up rested? Generally easy-going, mostly coping well? or Sleep badly, often tired, little energy? Irritable, touchy?			
SKIN, HAIR & NAILS Skin clear, sometimes spotty? Always spotty and clogged with grease? Smooth or rough & dry? Hair and nails glossy and strong, or dry & brittle			
OVERALL Trim ankles, waist and outline, or puffy areas, especially feet and wrist? Active muscles, zest for living, good posture, bright eyes?			

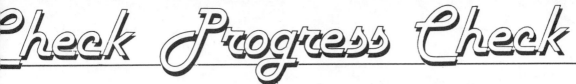

Decide what you want to aim for in a month, and then in a year. Remember to be sensible—if you set your sights too high, you're almost bound to fail. That could make you feel so miserable and anxious you give up altogether. So aim for weight loss of 2–5 pounds a week, no more, and a gradual change in your appearance and overall good health. You'll find a little patience pays dividends in the long term. If you do achieve your goal in $2\frac{1}{2}$ weeks every month, then perhaps you can be a little stricter, but don't go too far too fast.

Finally, fill in the columns as each week passes, judging how your general fitness is responding to good food and good exercise, and weighing yourself every week at the same time in the same clothes.

As you change to a new chart each month, keep the same goal for the year—think of the pleasure and delight you'll feel when the last two columns match up!

) WEEK	THIRD WEEK	FOURTH WEEK	A YEAR FROM NOW

Year Planner

Year Planner

1	**2**	**3**
4	**5**	**6**
7	**8**	**9**
10	**11**	**12**
13	**14**	**15**
16	**17**	**18**
19	**20**	**21**
22	**23**	**24**
25	**26**	**27**
28	**29**	**30**
31		

Begin a new year with a new plan; you *will* eat better, you *will* diet, you *will* exercise regularly. You *will* make every day count.

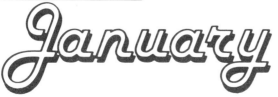

Here is your planner for the year, to help you get fit, stay healthy, and feel good all the time. Fill in your weight at least every two weeks – on the 1st and 15th of every month. Try to get some exercise every day, and make a note in the corner of the box. If you are counting calories, add up every evening and put the *real* number down, too. Then watch the pounds fall off.

1	2	3
4	5	6
7	8	9
10	11	12
13	14	15
16	17	18
19	20	21
22	23	24
25	26	27
28		

Wearing boots all winter is bad for feet; keep feet supple and flexible with extra exercise.

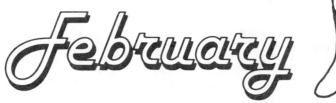

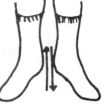

1	2	3
4	5	6
7	8	9
10	11	12
13	14	15
16	17	18
19	20	21
22	23	24
25	26	27
28	29	30
31	Biting winds roughen your face quickly; remember the moisturizer every day.	

March

1	2	3
4	5	6
7	8	9
10	11	12
13	14	15
16	17	18
19	20	21
22	23	24
25	26	27
28	29	30

Bikini weather soon — pick a diet and stick to it. Plant some new vegetables in the garden.

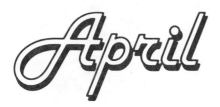

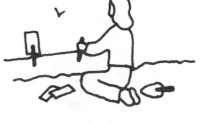

1	2	3
4	5	6
7	8	9
10	11	12
13	14	15
16	17	18
19	20	21
22	23	24
25	26	27
28	29	30
31	Plan your summer trip now. Make reservations, see about boarding the dog. Last-minute panics spoil the fun.	

May

$\boxed{1}$	2	3
4	5	6
7	8	9
10	11	12
13	14	$\boxed{15}$
16	17	18
19	20	21
22	23	24
25	26	27
28	29	30

Checking-up time. Give yourself a celebration salad if you lost weight. Check your eating habits if you didn't.

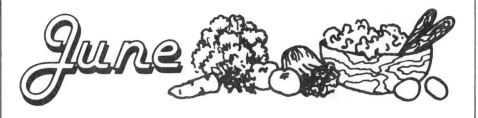

1	2	3
4	5	6
7	8	9
10	11	12
13	14	15
16	17	18
19	20	21
22	23	24
25	26	27
28	29	30
31		

Swimming is one of the best all-round sports; see that the children learn, too.

July

1	2	3
4	5	6
7	8	9
10	11	12
13	14	15
16	17	18
19	20	21
22	23	24
25	26	27
28	29	30
31	Sunburn can be painful; cover the back of your neck and hands when working outdoors.	

August

1	2	3
4	5	6
7	8	9
10	11	12
13	14	15
16	17	18
19	20	21
22	23	24
25	26	27
28	29	30

Time to make preserves, join a keep-fit class, take up a new hobby.

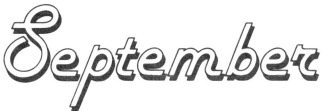

September

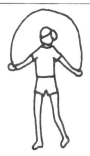

1	2	3
4	5	6
7	8	9
10	11	12
13	14	15
16	17	18
19	20	21
22	23	24
25	26	27
28	29	30
31		

Do home and garden renovations little by little; make sure you lift heavy loads properly.

October

1	2	3
4	5	6
7	8	9
10	11	12
13	14	15
16	17	18
19	20	21
22	23	24
25	26	27
28	29	30

Don't let loose sweaters hide spreading waistlines. Get enough vitamin D.

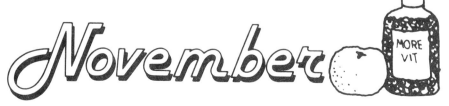

November

1	2	3
4	5	6
7	8	9
10	11	12
13	14	15
16	17	18
19	20	21
22	23	24
25	26	27
28	29	30
31		

Holiday preparations, a daily dozen to keep fit, half an hour a day just for you to relax. Merry Christmas!

December

Diet and Nutrition

Introduction

THE PLEASURE PRINCIPLE

It may seem unusual to start a section on good nutrition with a plea for delicious food on your table. But it's far too easy to fall into the trap of talking about nutrition as if it were only quantities of proteins, milligrams of numbered vitamins, units of minerals, and altogether a dry table of contents for the human body, used to correct deficiencies, control diseases and cure weight problems.

Nutrition is much more — at its best, it's the study of human beings in their environment, and how they are sustained and supported all through their lives by a healthy, functioning body.

Of course, for those who have to keep to a strict diet or a very restricted menu, there aren't many alternatives, and food becomes something to eat merely to stay alive and relatively well.

But for most of us, good food and good eating is a gift to ourselves three times a day, and enjoying what we eat is nutrition's gift to us. The relaxation and pleasure we feel during a good dinner actually helps the body to digest and assimilate food as quickly and smoothly as possible.

Remember the smell of fragrant soup bubbling with herbs and vegetables on a cold night? The aroma of freshly baked bread? The crunchy bite of crisp salad, the tang of oil and vinegar? Every time we respond to food in this way, our body has begun to manufacture the necessary enzymes, and the whole system gets ready to do its job in the best possible way.

There are other benefits from learning to enjoy food, too. Cooking is a time consuming part of every day, so it seems sensible to try and make it as easy and pleasant as possible. The easy part is learning the best way to prepare good food and our Cook's Guide should help you with that.

The pleasant aspects of cooking are the joys it can bring as a skill and a craft, and as something to share with the rest of the family, and with friends, too.

New recipes and unusual dishes make dinner time seem more of an adventure, and with a whole world of recipes to choose from, you could probably cook for a year without ever repeating the same dish. Equally, simple natural foods taste good; no matter how many times there are crisp apples and cheese on the table, they will always be welcome, and always taste slightly different.

Children should enjoy cooking and preparing food, too. They love to bake gingerbread men and carefully swirl meringue kisses onto the rice paper. Most children are so delighted with the fun of creating delicious things that they will be willing and useful helpers for many of the duller chores.

Finally, an extra bonus — cooking can be a therapy, a way of pausing for a moment or two in the day's frantic rush to shell or cut and arrange in lovely patterns. Food should be a pleasure for the eye as well as the palate, and the act of making a dish look fresh and appetizing is often a good way of relaxing. If you are really upset, then baking bread can be the answer – kneading dough hard and punching it down over and over again may make the bread take a little longer to rise than usual, but it will lighten your heart wonderfully.

All of this doesn't mean that food should become the be-all and end-all of our day. A gourmet who appreciates fine food is not a glutton who gobbles down endless platters. We must not confuse quality with quantity, encouraging reluctant guests to eat more than they would like, as if we are going to be judged by how much food is actually on the table when we get up after dinner.

Eating can be a real delight, but it must never be a substitute for living or loving. We should regard it as a way of sustaining life and a part of life, a nourishing ingredient for ourselves and our families, which we can serve every day with pride, and with pleasure. The joy of food, certainly, and food for joy, always.

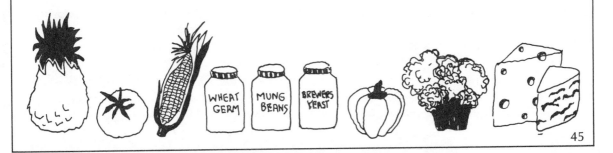

The New Nutrition

A DIET REVOLUTION

What you eat matters, because first rate nutrition is probably the single most important factor in gaining health and keeping it. The foods you eat form the foundation of every cell in your body and when they are the right foods, they contribute to sound tissues, organs, muscles and skin. Your foundation is firm, your energy level is high, your body strong, your mind clear and your emotions stable. But when the foundation is shaky as a result of living on wrong foods – those that cannot supply all the important factors your body needs for both cell building and day-to-day living – then you are more susceptible to illness of every kind.

Recent scientific studies of the relationship between nutrition and health in most of the countries of the world have turned up important evidence indicating that certain diseases which have become widespread in the western world such as obesity, dental problems, peptic ulcers, coronary heart disease, diverticulosis and diabetes have many of their roots in the type of foods we eat and the way they are processed and prepared. This has brought about a new surge of interest in the powers of nutrition and thrown the whole subject of what we should eat and how we can get the best health value out of foods into a new light.

Years ago, long lists of 'minimum daily requirements' were drawn up and it was implied that one's diet should be carefully planned around them. We knew just exactly how much of a particular vitamin was necessary every day in order to prevent the symptoms of certain serious illnesses and that was enough. It was never stated how much one needed to be as fit and healthy as possible, but only how little one could take and still not become blatantly ill. Such minimum requirements were useful but limiting, a slightly mechanistic way of thinking that implied that so long as you got so many calories, such and such milligrams of each vitamin, and so many grams of protein each day, it didn't matter how.

Imagine a scrumptious pink ice cream, filled with chemically made vitamins, and 'fortified' with protein – you'd have the 'perfect food'. Then why bother with foods like fresh fruits and vegetables, fish, meat, and poultry, whole grain and cereals, which take far longer to prepare than opening a carton of ice cream and were more of a nuisance to buy and store? The idea sounded good except that when adults and children lived on a diet made up mostly from 'foods' fortified with vitamins and protein, it didn't work. Teeth decayed, kids got fat, and governments voiced concern about the low levels of fitness in the youth in some of the richest countries in the world.

It's obvious that these highly processed, fortified foods, delicious as they might be, are not the answer to basic nutritional needs, no matter how much they supposedly provide in the way of required vitamins, calories, proteins, carbohydrates and fats.

Today, there is a new attitude about the foods we eat and how best to use them to preserve health. Where yesterday's scientists thought all we needed was a certain amount of vitamin C plus all the other nutrients, today's biochemists, doctors and nutritionists believe we need not only the minimum daily requirements of nutrients, but also specific kinds of foods, in a proper balance, processed, prepared and served to preserve their highest potential for health. Because other as-yet unidentified substances in food may contribute to keeping one fit, good nutrition depends on a far greater range of factors than we first thought. Far from being sure of everything, the present breed of nutritionists are all too ready to admit that there is still much we do not know about how food affects health.

The new nutritionists are vigorously exploring two questions which are absolutely vital to today's world. First, how can nutrition be employed to help protect against certain damaging effects of environmental pollution such as from chemicals in the water we drink and the air we breathe? Second, how can we use nutrition to promote *positive* health rather than merely lack of disease. Perhaps this is the most practical result. We know now that everyone has a potential for health and fitness that is usually far greater than they realize, and good eating habits are one of the most important keys for unlocking it. Two things are needed. First, information. Second, action. The following section supplies the information; the action is up to you.

FOODS TO CHOOSE FROM

Wholegrain bread
Wholewheat pasta (spaghetti, macaroni, green lasagne)
Brown rice (long or short grain)
100% wholegrain flour (wheat, rye, corn, soya)
Old-fashioned porridge (from whole cracked wheat or oats)
Wholegrain cereals without sugar
Fresh vegetables (leafy green, tubers and bulbs)
Frozen vegetables
Fresh fruits and unsweetened juices
Frozen fruits (without sugar)
Meat
Fish
Poultry
Eggs
Cheese
Milk
Yogurt
Butter or margarine
Vegetable oils
Herbs and spices

FOODS TO AVOID

Note: (If you must eat many of these very often, make sure you get added bran)

White bread, rolls and pastries
White pasta (spaghetti, macaroni, etc)
White rice
White flour
Most crackers
Sugar coated cereals
Cereals not made from whole grain

WHAT IS FOOD AND HOW DO WE USE IT?

What is food? Food is, quite simply, fuel. Just as an automobile uses combustion for energy, humans utilize food to keep their engines going. And just as impure fuel and oil adversely affect the running of an engine, bad eating habits will make humans (and particularly *growing* humans) unhealthy. This section, *Diet and Nutrition*, will discuss not only what food is, but what *good* food is; not simply how we use it, but how we should use it for our greatest benefit.

A Crash Course in Digestion

Every particle of food that we put into our mouths, from an ice cream cone on a hot day to a complete, seven course Chinese dinner, is subject to a remarkably complex chemical process which involves just about every muscle and nerve in our body, including the brain.

As soon as food is put into the mouth, a message is sent to the brain requesting the glands to begin secreting *saliva*. (Sometimes only the smell or even the thought of a delicious food can stimulate the saliva glands.) The *teeth* begin masticating or chewing the food – this grinding serving two purposes. First, it prepares the food for its tour through the rest of the digestive system, and second it begins to digest the carbohydrates. (The other food substances are worked on in the stomach and the intestines.) The *tongue* helps the food down towards the throat where the *epiglottis* comes into action, closing off the wind pipe and directing the food toward the *stomach*.

The tube connecting the mouth and throat to the stomach is called the *esophagus*. The esophagus is equipped with tiny nerve endings that instigate a muscle-like action called *peristalsis* that helps push the food along the tube toward the stomach.

When the food reaches the stomach, hydrochloric acid and the enzyme pepsin begin to break down the proteins, turning them into simpler materials called amino acids. Alcohol is the only foodstuff that the stomach wall allows to escape; all other foodstuffs are sent on to the intestines for final digestion.

After the food gets as far as the *duodenum* or the first ten inches of the *small intestine*, the really complicated chemical breakdowns begin. In the stomach, the food has been reacted upon by acids. These acids also activate the intestinal hormones which stimulate the *liver* and the *pancreas* to secrete *bile* and *pancreatic juice* into the intestine. These juices and the intestine's own juices are alkaline and neutralize the acids collected in the stomach. Also the intestine's enzymes act on the food to break it down to the point where it is almost ready to yield its nutrients into the system.

Once all these juices are activated, it takes four to eight hours for all foods to be digested. Peristalsis comes into the act again, pushing the food through the small intestine. As the food moves along, millions of microscopic protrusions called *villi* transfer the usable food nutrients from the intestine to the blood and lymph systems.

Finally, what's left of the food remains in the large intestine for another 10 to 12 hours losing water. Then, the bacteria work to decay the remains which are passed on through the colon as waste.

This is an extremely simplified discussion of the very complicated digestive system. Our bodies, as you can see, are truly very like engines and the food (which is turned into chemicals) is the fuel that keeps that engine going. Because digestion is one of humanity's most fundamental processes, one is tempted to say it is almost philosophical in nature. It's the Biblical 'You reap what you sow' story. In other words, the better the food is that we put into our bodies, the better our bodies will work at digesting that food.

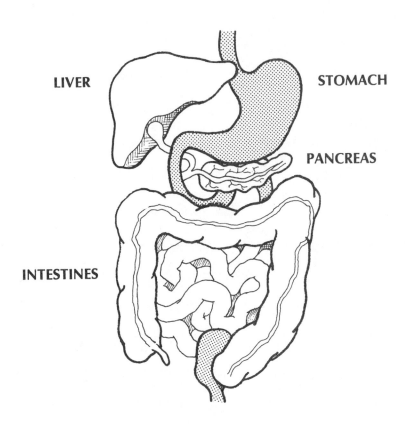

LIVER

STOMACH

PANCREAS

INTESTINES

What Is Food?

A Crash Course in Nutrition

Food is basically made up of a number of basic elements: carbohydrates, proteins, fats, vitamins, minerals, certain vitamin-like trace elements, and water.

Carbohydrates (sugars and starches), as has been pointed out, are the foods most quickly digested. Because of the speedy breakdown by the body, carbohydrates are used primarily for quick energy. They are, perhaps unfortunately for those with an overweight problem, the largest single component aside from water in an average daily diet, comprising slightly over one half of our calorie intake each day.

Proteins are extremely complex substances made up of many substructures called amino acids. Protein is a constituent of every living cell, plant and animal, and they are used by the body for the growth and repair of every body tissue. Although all nutrients are of equal importance and a diet lacking in any would be insufficient and unhealthy, proteins are of utmost importance in the functioning of the body. Without them, life would be virtually impossible.

Fats are primarily used by the body for reserve energy. They are stored, ready to be called on for energy, when a diet is short of carbohydrates and proteins. It is not difficult to deduce that the best — and perhaps the only — way to lose body fat is to reduce the intake of carbohydrates, proteins, and of course, food fats, so that the storehouse of body fat can be absorbed. (To put it more simply, the best weight loss diet is to eat less!)

In the 19th century, nutritional studies began to show that the body could not live on just the basic elements of carbohydrates, fats, proteins, and water. It was then discovered that *minerals* were of vital importance in human nutrition. Many minerals are used by the body, with calcium (used mainly for strengthening bone material) and iron (especially for women) being two that people think of most readily. Others of importance include phosphorus, potassium, sulfur, sodium, zinc, copper, and iodine.

Minerals are used for a number of intricate systems, including maintaining the acid-base balance of enzymes, as catalysts for certain biological reactions, maintaining the water balance, transmitting nerve impulses, and regulating muscle contractions.

Vitamins were the last group of dietary essentials to be recognized by scientists, perhaps because they are needed by the body in such minute quantities. Vitamins are organic substances that perform a specific metabolic function (depending upon the vitamin), and as a result are essential to the diet.

If one nutrient should be considered more important than any other, it is *water*, yet because it is so often taken for granted, it is often overlooked in a discussion of nutrition. (Note later, in the discussion of the various diets, that the importance of water is mentioned consistently.) A person can live for many days without food and sometimes for years without certain basic vitamins or minerals, but he would survive for only a few days without water.

Like proteins, water is a constitutent of every living cell, making up about 60% of total body weight. Water serves a number of purposes in the digestive process. It acts as a solvent for the nutrients and for the hormones secreted by the glands and carries them by way of the blood and lymph system to all the cells of the body. It also collects waste products from the cells and carries them away to be eliminated.

Water within cells works to help synthesize new material while water in such fluids as saliva lubricates food facilitating its passage through the digestive system. Studies also show that water plays a role in the metabolism of the nutrients with the conclusion that lack of water slows up the metabolic process. Finally, water regulates body temperature.

It is beyond the scope of this book to go into a detailed accounting of precisely which elements are contained in which food groups. Suffice to say that each of the four groups were chosen because each made unique contribution to the diet and each is essential. However, other considerations such as calories or certain vitamin deficiencies should also be taken into account. For example, some green vegetables such as lima beans have far more calories than others such as string beans. One member of your family may be allergic to or require more of a specific vitamin or mineral, in which case foods containing these elements should be avoided or used more frequently depending, of course, on the problem. Any basic textbook on nutrition can guide you – or consult your doctor if such a problem exists.

VITAMIN SUPPLEMENTS

Vitamin supplements continue to be a source of controversy in the health world. The traditional view is that the ordinary diet in the Western countries is more than adequate to meet all known vitamin requirements. The vitamin-takers point to reports which link larger-than-normal doses with the prevention of many serious diseases, as well as the common cold. In fact, there seems to be no simple way to make a decision. We are such complicated animals that although we can see fairly easily when there is a very large deficiency (scurvy which comes from too little Vitamin C, anaemia from too little Vitamin B and iron) it is much harder to pinpoint the amount of any vitamin you may need in order to feel your very best all the time.

Perhaps the best way of making a choice is to try taking a good vitamin and mineral supplement for six months, and judging for yourself if it has made a difference in how you feel, and how you look.

But one word of warning – do be careful about taking very large doses of individual vitamins. Most of them are synergestic; that is, they work together in the body and depend on each other to do their job well. This is particularly true of the B complex group. It is better for your overall health to take a really complete supplement which includes everything your body needs rather than pick out one or two fashionable letters which are the latest miracle workers.

NOTE FOR CHARTS: The Recommended Dietary Allowance is a basic guideline for good nutrition. We show the average adult requirement, or where there is a wide variation, the range from children to adults. Pregnant and breast-feeding women should take the highest amounts, plus a little extra. Check with your doctor for particular needs; we are all a little different.

NUTRIENT	R.D.A.	FOODS RICH IN	DAILY ALLOWANCE IN FOOD
VITAMIN A	800–4000 IU	Dark green leafy vegetables, deep orange vegetables, and fruits, some meats, some milk, eggs	1 cup cooked carrots $\frac{1}{2}$ cantaloupe melon 1 cup cooked beet greens 1 persimmon 1 raw sweet red pepper 1 apricot 1 peach 1 tomato raw $\frac{1}{2}$ grapefruit 1 large egg 1 ounce Cheddar cheese 1 cup whole milk
VITAMIN D	400 IU For Children only	Dairy products, milk, some in egg yolks, butter, SUNLIGHT	4 8-ounce glasses of whole milk 12 large egg yolks 14 tablespoons butter
VITAMIN E	9–15 IU	Oils, nuts, grains, some vegetables, fruits, chocolate; but not in large quantities, so you'd need a lot of bulk Grains contribute, but need a lot of bulk to be sole supply Vegetables are a little better Fruits poor except for:	9–15 tablespoons olive oil 2 tablespoons safflower oil BUT NOTE: peanut and sesame oil, only 3 IU per tablespoon slice wholemeal enriched bread 5 cups cornmeal 9 cups raw brown rice $\frac{3}{4}$ lb beet top greens 5–6 large stalks broccoli 18 Brussels sprouts 10 leeks $\frac{2}{3}$ lb spinach $1\frac{1}{2}$ sweet potatoes *Wild* blackberries, 8.6 a cup, but note, 1.5 a cup cultivated!
VITAMIN C	45 mgs	Fresh fruit & vegetables (not only oranges, but is stable in citrus fruit, & may be lost easily in storage and cooking of other foods)	1 orange $\frac{1}{2}$ grapefruit $\frac{1}{2}$ cantaloupe melon 4 bananas 2 tomatoes 2 cups raw spinach 1 stalk broccoli 3–4 Brussels sprouts 2 boiled potatoes with jacket $\frac{2}{3}$ cup cauliflower

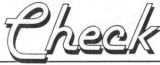

Vitamin Check

NUTRIENT	R.D.A.	FOODS RICH IN	DAILY ALLOWANCE IN FOOD
VITAMIN K		Leafy dark green vegetables, egg yolks,	amount required so small that a normal good-health diet will supply enough
FOLACIN (Folic Acid)	400 mgs	Legumes, vegetables, fruits, juices	$1^3/_4$ cup dry garbazo (chick peas) $1^3/_4$ cup dry kidney beans 6 stalks broccoli 15 large Brussels sprouts 9 beets $^1/_2$ lb spinach $2^1/_2$ cups fresh orange juice $1^1/_3$ tablespoons brewer's yeast $1^2/_3$ tablespoons dried yeast
NIACIN (Nicotinic Acid)	13 mgs	Soybeans, greens, beans and grains	$^3/_4$ cup soybeans uncooked 2 cups cottage cheese 3 cups fresh peas 3 cups lentils 8 tablespoons peanuts 4–5 large eggs 16 tablespoons sunflower seeds 10 oz Cheddar cheese
RIBOFLAVIN B2	1.2 mgs	Milk, leafy green vegetables, beans	2 cups cottage cheese 3 cups low fat yogurt $2^2/_3$ cups whole milk 4 stalks broccoli 5 portions camembert
THIAMIN B1	1.0 mgs	Yeasts, whole grains, legumes	1 tablespoon brewer's yeast $2^1/_2$ cups fresh green peas cooked 8 oz raw barley 5 large oranges $2^1/_2$ whole avocado pears 10 stalks broccoli
B6 Pyridoxine	2.0 mgs	Whole grains, beans, some vegetables but destroyed by heat & processing	$2^1/_2$ lb raw spinach $3^1/_2$ bananas 2 cups dry lentils 4 cantaloupes 8 cups raw green peas
B12	3.0 mgs	Milk and most milk products, except for butter	$1^1/_2$ cups cottage cheese 3 cups whole or skim milk 3 eggs 6 oz Swiss & cream cheeses 12 oz Cheddar cheese

NOTE: All allowances given are for the full daily amount from one source only.

MINERALS	RECOMMENDED AMOUNT	SOURCES: PORTIONS
SODIUM – SODIUM CHLORIDE (Table Salt)	Basic eating with no salt added will still give you five times the amount you need, which is about $1/5$ teaspoonful a day.	
CALCIUM	Teenagers and Pregnant women 1,200 mg Adults 800 mg	20 cups blackberries $1^1/_2$ pints butter-milk or whole milk 4 oz cheddar cheese 3 oz Swiss cheese 24 oz cottage cheese $1^1/_2$ lbs lobster meat 1 lb macaroni and cheese $1^1/_2$ pints whole or skim milk 5 tablespoons black molasses 8 pancakes with butter & syrup 4 cups of rice pudding 4 cups of cooked rhubarb 7 oz of sardines OR 350 oz of tuna fish 4 small cartons of plain yoghurt 4 cups cooked greens
IRON	Teenagers and pregnant women 80 mg Adult males 10 mg Women 18 mg	2 lbs of almonds 10 avocados 2–3 cups cooked dried beans $1^1/_2$ lbs hamburger meat $1^1/_4$ cups enriched farma $1^1/_2$ lbs clams & oysters (shelled) OR 5 lbs crabmeat 7 oz kidney or liver 6 tablespoons black molasses 10 oz turkey meat

NOTE: Recommended amounts are generally higher than absolute minimum required.

Check Mineral Check

MINERALS	RECOMMENDED AMOUNT	SOURCES: PORTIONS
MAGNESIUM	Teenagers 350–400 mg Adults 300 mg Pregnant women 450 mg	1 cup dried beans 12 cups cooked macaroni 6 oz dried buckwheat (kasha) 12 tablespoons peanut butter 19 tablespoons sesame seeds 1 lb beet top greens 21 brussel sprouts 120 mushrooms $^3/_4$ lb spinach 30 apples or peaches 6 avocados 6 cups blackberries 4 pints whole, skim or butter-milk 2 lbs dandelion greens Whole greens, nuts, beans and green leafed vegetables.
IODINE	Males 130 mcg to 110 as older Females 115 mcg to 80 as older	Trace only, in most vegetables, usually added to table salt
PHOSPHORUS	As above	4 tablespoons pumpkin seeds $2^1/_3$ cups cottage cheese 3 cups cooked red beans $1^1/_2$ pints milk
ZINC	Teenagers and adults 15 mg Pregnant women 20 mg	7 cups of garbanzo beans 7 cups of cooked green peas 10 oz of soya flour 5 cups cooked spinach

55

GETTING STARTED ON GOOD HEALTH

Many homemakers who become aware of the basic principles of good nutrition and the important part that food plays in overall fitness are then faced with a big problem: how do you convert a family used to eating large quantities of over-processed convenience foods to healthier eating habits? This is not difficult to solve provided you have just a little patience at the beginning and plan your meals well.

Think of a family of four. At the doctor's request the husband is on a diet that is low in cholesterol and fat. He is also advised not to eat lots of sugar. Concerned about her waistline, the wife has put herself on a calorie-controlled diet to lose a few pounds. One child, a boy of eight, will eat only hamburgers or chicken with potatoes and gooey desserts. The other child, a teenage daughter is 'hip', into natural foods, meditation and vegetarianism. What does the cook do?

One solution: a chicken in the oven roasted along with three potatoes in their jackets for the children and the husband, steamed broccoli, a large raw vegetable salad and fresh fruit for dessert.

At the table Father eats the chicken, a baked potato with natural yogurt and chopped chives on it instead of butter or margarine, broccoli and salad. The young child has the same but with butter on his baked potato. The wife eats everything except the potato. The teenage daughter eats everything but

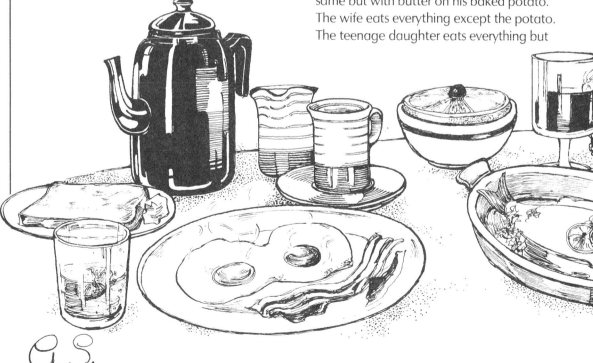

G.S.

the chicken and sprinkles some grated cheese on her baked potato for extra protein. Another night the whole family might have a pasta dish with a rich vegetable sauce which Mother eats over an omelette instead. The permutations are endless, and all the menus in this section suggest basic dishes which can easily be adapted to individual needs.

In raising the level of 'nutrition-consciousness' of your family, go slowly. Avoid long discussions of how bad 'bad' foods are for health. Instead simply introduce new nutritious items to the table in small quantities. When you do put a new food on the table don't make a big fuss, and don't even mention its vitamin content. Concentrate on the good taste. An 'eat-it-because-it's-good-for-you' tone is sure to alienate most of the family.

Children are also enthusiastic bread makers once they know how and usually are very proud of their creative efforts. To change from white packaged bread to wholegrain, try making your own. Homemade bread is always a winner. Begin by using unbleached white flour; then gradually each week add a little more wholegrain flour to the recipe.

A teenager (or anyone else!) who is passionate about ecology and natural foods can be a great ally in preparing and serving foods that win over the rest of the family to a better lifestyle. When all the family is involved in the kitchen, making dishes of all kinds, experimenting, tasting, the greater enthusiasts they become for well-prepared fresh nourishing foods. And once they taste the difference between the pre-cooked packaged heat-in-a-minute dinner and the beautifully prepared home cooking that they have made your battle is won.

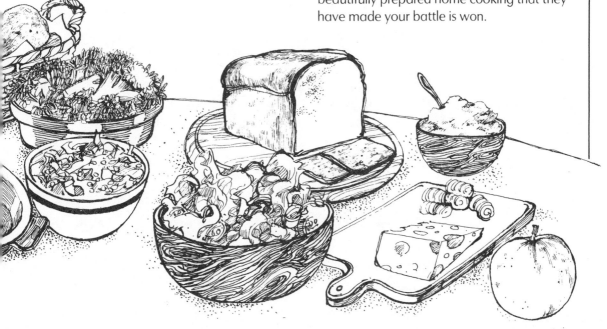

THE GOOD HEALTH KITCHEN

Good food and good health can go together in everyone's daily life. Don't throw away all those lovely cookbooks you've collected over the years. Almost every recipe can be easily adapted to give more nutritional value *and* better, more natural-tasting dishes at the same time. Even if you are not on a diet, the following hints will help to retain the vitamin and mineral content in the food, lower the quantity of unnecessary fats, sugars and salts on your plate, and let the fresh taste of your food make mealtimes a pleasure for the entire family.

SALT AND SUGAR

Try using less sugar and salt than a recipe calls for, and increasing the quantity of herbs if you need a sharper taste. Both sweetness and spice are a matter of habit – we expect cakes and desserts to be sugary and it's amazing how much less can be used if you reduce the amount gradually. Accustom your family to more natural sweetness. Salt is also often over-generously provided; try using very little or none while you are cooking, and adjust the seasoning at the table. Don't worry about not getting enough – most foods have quite a lot of natural salt (and sugar) and we eat every day at least ten times the amount of both seasonings that our bodies need to stay healthy. Experiment with quantities gradually, though, to avoid sudden changes.

VEGETABLES

Good health begins with basic ingredients – you've taken the trouble to choose fresh food, full of goodness and vitamins, so don't ruin it with poor preparation and bad health habits. That means careful storage when you get the food home; that bowl of fruit left out for days on end may make the house look like an illustration from a magazine, but you're letting the vitamins fade away in the light and warmth of the room. After three days at normal room temperature, fruit and vegetables may have lost up to 70 % of their Vitamin A, C and D. Store foods carefully, in a dark cool food cupboard, or in the refrigerator. Meat and poultry and all perishable goods should be kept in the refrigerator for best conservation and longest storage life.

Don't waste good vitamins by throwing away carrot tops, beet tops, cabbage hearts, or other greens. They make delicious vegetables when steamed for a few moments with a few fresh herbs and a bit of butter. The not-so-perfect bits are good for stock, or they will make a thick, nourishing vegetable soup.

MEAT

The leanest cuts of meat are usually the most expensive, but even the best steak can contain quite a lot of fat hidden in the cells.

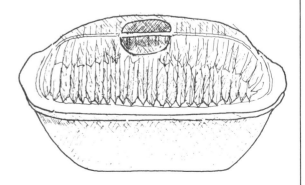

58

Cooking in a clay pot is best for lean meat only. Cut away all the visible fat and gristle, especially from long-cooking stewing and casserole meats. Poultry, particularly duck, geese and capon, often has layers of fat under the skin and in the dark-meat sections. Cut that away too. Of course, if you do trim the meat carefully, half the quantity gets thrown away. Sometimes it is just as economical to buy more expensive cuts and serve smaller portions. Not a bad idea in any case, because most of us eat too much, and especially too much meat. Increase the amount of vegetables instead; it will make a much more balanced meal.

BUTTERS AND FATS

There has been much controversy about unsaturated and saturated fats, butter or oils, hard fats or soft fats. Medical opinion varies, but one thing they are all certain of is that we eat more fat than we need. Use smaller quantities, especially in meat and vegetable dishes. (It's harder to change the amount in baking recipes without adjusting the rest of the ingredients.) When you fry, make sure the fat is hot enough to seal the food immediately. A fat thermometer is a useful investment, because instead of guessing when the fat is ready, you'll know the exact second. This means less cooking time, less chance of burning the fat and having to throw it away, and crisper, more palatable food.

COOKING

Get into the habit of steaming vegetables instead of boiling them. Steaming keeps all the vitamins and minerals inside the food instead of in the water to be thrown away. A steamer doesn't cost much. Buy an adjustable wire basket on legs that can sit inside any saucepan. Add just enough water to make the steam rise and cook the vegetables. Don't overcook. Vegetables taste so much better when they are slightly crisp and chewy instead of mushy, water-sodden lumps.

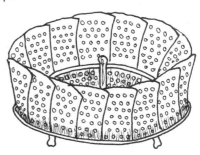

Almost all recipes which call for boiling can be adapted to steaming. This includes fish and even meat, although since it takes much longer to cook watch the pot carefully to see the water doesn't boil dry.

POTS AND PANS

Non-stick pans are a great boon to the careful cook, since it means food can be sautéed and fried with a minimum of fat. Many lean-looking meats do contain hidden fat, and this should be poured off as often as necessary. Non-stick pans can replace the classic frying pan in most recipes; the new coatings are very tough and shouldn't require special tools.

There are also heavy saucepans and casseroles available which cook on low heats with very little added liquid. This is always an advantage as the nutrition stays in the food, instead of being left in the oil or water.

The oriental wok is another useful buy for the careful cook. The special rounded base means that all the ingredients are cooked quickly in the middle of the pan. You'll need much less oil, and probably less seasoning as well.

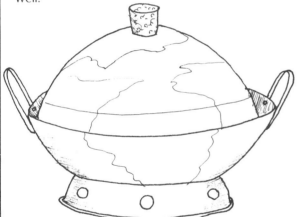

herbs and spices, one of the oldest pieces of equipment in the world is still unbeatable – a pestle and mortar. There is just no better way to crush peppercorns and seeds at the last minute, so all the aroma is still there when you add the spice to the food. Antique wooden sets are lovely to look at, but modern ones made of composition or glass are actually better, because the wood absorbs oils and odors from the spice, and may transfer a bit of your crushed ginger to the next night's cummin or coriander seed.

When you have a pestle, then buy your spices in small quantities so that they are as fresh as possible - this is one case where economy-size packets are for restaurants only. And buy whole spices when you can – you'll never really appreciate what they can do for your cooking until you try the difference between dried-out bits of tasteless garlic and freshly-crushed cloves prepared a moment or two before being used. And a moment or two is all it takes.

SPECIAL EQUIPMENT

Pressure cookers are a useful aid to the good cook, since they make it possible to cook inexpensive cuts of meat in a very short time. They are a form of high-pressure steamer, so you get the benefits of steaming instead of boiling as well. With today's interest in food gardening, pressure cookers are also useful for preserving bottled fruits and vegetables, and sterilizing jam and marmalade jars. Buy a good solid model, and follow directions carefully.

For the cook who develops an interest in

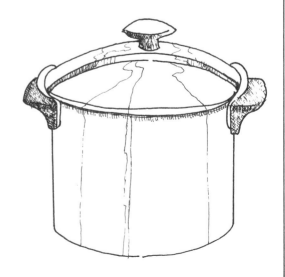

There are dozens of new appliances available today, as modern as the pestle and mortar are old. Some are passing fancies, more gimmicky than useful, some are limited to one kind of usefulness, and whether you buy them or not depends very much on your individual family. But there are two electric cooking aids which are so important to the health-minded cook that they are worth considering as basic as a set of good knives, and better for your over-all nutrition than any frying pan; a blender or liquidizer, and one of the new food processors. Both are worth saving up for.

The blender has been around for a few years, and with it comes the perfect way to get every bit of taste and nourishment from fresh fruits and vegetables. It will make purées and juices from raw food, whip up healthy delicious drinks from milk and other ingredients, make gravies and sauces from cooked vegetables so that you don't need to add flour or thickenings, and do a hundred and one other jobs quickly and easily. Buy the biggest you can afford, so you can handle food in largish batches, and try to find one that unscrews at the base so that you can get out every last bit of mixture.

Food processors are quite new, and still expensive, but they have literally revolutionized home preparation, especially of salads and fresh vegetables. They are a combination of blender and mixer, with powerful motors that whirl the blades around so fast an entire cabbage can be shredded in literally seconds. The makings of a mixed salad for twenty people would take a few minutes as most, including evenly sliced raw

mushrooms, rings of green pepper, slivered onions and shredded carrots.

Fresh nuts and seeds are ground to powder in seconds, indigestable cabbage hearts turn into tender shreds for steaming, raw meat becomes a light and fluffy paté you can almost eat without cooking, and all in a single bowl easy to wash out, self-contained in a small unit so it fits into even miniature kitchens. Practically all of the tedious preparation that makes busy cooks reach for convenience foods has been eliminated. It will help you change your ideas and your menus in a way hard to believe until you own one.

Freezers
Freezing is a boon to the good cook no matter what sort of diet the family is used to – it preserves fresh food more quickly than any other form of storage, and keeps as much of the vitamins as possible in the original state. Meat, vegetables, bread, desserts – almost everything can be prepared for freezing, and it makes it possible to plan ahead whenever the garden is overflowing with fresh food. But do use your freezer properly – get a good instruction book to remind you about blanching and storage time – not all freezers have the same temperature control, and a freezer thermometer is a good extra to make sure it is working properly.

Above all, label whatever you put in – you may think that it's easy to see that spinach is green, and lamb chops are pink, but in two or three months both will be shapeless white bundles.

Natural Foods

EATING NATURALLY

Natural foods taste great: red and green salads fresh from the garden, wholegrain bread and fruity jam, a chicken with real chicken taste – no wonder a return to natural foods is one of the most important trends we've witnessed in recent years.

Modern progress in preservation, production and processing has certainly added an enormous variety of trouble-free foods to our menus. But it is not all a miracle. Some methods are potentially dangerous to health. Gases are used to ripen and preserve fruits and vegetables. Chemical sprays are applied and fertilizers are spread with alarming casualness over our farm lands.

Such substances and chemical compounds may have long-term effects which no one yet understands. We now consume the equivalent of two to five pounds of these additives per person per year, about 10 to 40 tablets a day, taken year in year out. And consumption is going up every week as we buy more and more convenience foods.

Of course, it is important not to become so anti-manufactured food that we reject everything that has been processed in any way. Much of the processing, such as the milling of whole wheat to make flour is very useful. And many food additives have a worthwhile and serious purpose. They make sure that those of us who live a long way from agricultural areas will have unspoiled, fresh tasting food without risking illness or even death which could occur as a result of poor storage or rancidity. After all, life was not all golden in the 'Golden Past':

tuberculosis from the milk of infected cows, trichinosis from pork. Green potatoes contain solanon, rhubarb leaves are poisonous, and even healthy spinach can be toxic! So we should keep a sense of proportion and encourage research that concentrates on improving present testing methods. Too many additives are tested only by themselves. Chemicals are known to interact with each other in a living organism. Safe even when taken in large doses on their own, some chemicals, when combined with other chemicals in food, might be very harmful indeed. This is one reason many people are interested in learning about a more natural way of life, growing their own food in healthy soil, and eating it in the primary state – raw or lightly cooked, using the skins of fruits and the green tops of vegetables as much as possible.

But unfortunately some campaigners for natural foods become fanatical about it. 'Natural' gets confused with 'health foods', and anything bought in a health food store must be healthier and better for you than products from your local supermarket. This is completely untrue. There are over-priced and even over-processed foods on the shelves of some health food stores, too, containing large quantities of sugar, and brown sugar is not much better than white. Others may be good for you but sell for outrageously high prices. Wholegrain flour, beans, etc may be much cheaper in a supermarket. There are also excellent suppliers of natural foods in bulk that can be purchased by mail at very reasonable prices.

In other words, shop carefully and read the labels, no matter where you are.

The Life-Long Diet

BASIC GUIDELINES

Since there are no restrictions on this diet, use it to your advantage to explore all the wonderful foods available. A week's worth of menus based on the four basic food groups are provided to stimulate your creativity. But go on from there and enjoy yourself.

Choose much of what you eat from foods in their raw or natural state: vegetables for salads, fruits, grains like brown rice and whole wheat bread and lean cuts of meat and fresh fish. This way you will get the highest complement of all the essential nutriments.

Don't be misled by claims of so-called 'miracle foods' such as 'enriched' or 'fortified' foods that give everybody everything. There are *no* real miracles at the supermarket. Stick to basic principles and basic foods.

Prepare as many of your foods as possible from scratch, relying on fresh herbs and natural ingredients. Cooking can be great fun as many people are rediscovering after years of relying on pre-cooked, packaged instant products. Good cooking can be a highly creative activity that brings great rewards in good health and the bonus of unusual dishes and delicious meals that everyone enjoys.

Alcohol uses up B complex vitamins and other important nutrients which your cells need to protect them from damage and which your whole body needs for continuing health. Keep hard liquor to a minimum. A glass of wine often relaxes tension and stimulates the palate, but too much has the opposite effect.

In addition, here are a few thoughts about basic nutrition and good eating:

● Familiarize yourself with some of the more exotic international cuisines such as Chinese, Japanese, Indian, or Mexican.

● Collect cookbooks and utensils. Try to make a special dinner one or two nights a month, or a special recipe once a week.

● Experiment with unusual meats such as chicken livers or many types of fish that are now more readily available.

● Learn to cook using as many fresh foods, particularly vegetables, as you can. They taste better than canned or packaged goods and are often cheaper.

● Decrease the amount of fat and sugar in your diet. Cut off all visible fat from meat and use less butter. Replace sweet desserts with fruits. All fat and most sugar required for the normal diet is there naturally without being added to dishes.

● Don't worry too much about the details. Try to develop good habits for choosing and cooking foods and then forget about it. Don't talk constantly about what you should or should not eat. Of course, it's important, but it must not become an obsession. There is far more to a healthy, happy life than concentrating all one's attention on food. Get out and live.

Life-long Menus

Here are two weeks of menus for the average adult family. Children should also drink four glasses of milk a day, and if you have no weight problem, you can add two cups for yourself. Always make the soups with skimmed milk instead of water for added protein, and choose any snacks from a variety of fresh fruit and cheese.

FIRST WEEK

BREAKFAST	Orange Juice Bacon and Tomato Wholewheat Toast
LUNCH	Cream of Vegetable Soup with Grated Cheese French Bread
DINNER	Fish Fillets on Leaf Spinach Red Cabbage and Chestnuts Creamed Potatoes Apples, Pears and Nuts

BREAKFAST	Cold Cereal, Sliced Bananas Milk or Cream
LUNCH	Raisin, Carrot and Walnut Salad Marinated Green Beans
DINNER	Curried Meat Balls Lentil Purée, Plain Rice Cucumber and Yoghurt Salad Ice Cream with Apricot Sauce

BREAKFAST	Fruit Juice Fried Eggs and Tomatoes
LUNCH	Cottage Cheese with Fresh Fruit Salad
DINNER	Chicken and Mushroom Gravy Herb Dumplings Brussels Sprouts, Carrots Cheese Board

SECOND WEEK

BREAKFAST	Sliced Fresh Fruit with Flaked Bran and Cream
LUNCH	Chicken Salad Mayonnaise Green Pepper Salad
DINNER	Baked Noodles and Cottage Cheese Green Salad, French Dressing Redcurrant Pudding

BREAKFAST	$^1/_2$ Grapefruit Sausage and Tomato
LUNCH	Mushroom and Barley Soup Granary Bread
DINNER	Fish Pie with Potato Topping Broccoli Corn and Red Peppers $^1/_2$ Melon (Honeydew or Cantaloupe)

BREAKFAST	Kippered Herring Fillets Wholewheat Toast
LUNCH	Stuffed Eggs with Mustard Green Salad
DINNER	Liver and Onions Fried Potatoes Cucumber and Radish Salad Fresh Fruit Salad with Coconut

FIRST WEEK

BREAKFAST	¹/₂ Grapefruit Oatmeal Porridge with Honey
LUNCH	Country Vegetable Soup French Bread
DINNER	Oven-baked Fish, Mustard Sauce Sliced Potato Casserole Pickled Beet Salad Plum Pudding with Cream

BREAKFAST	Orange Juice Pancakes and Tiny Sausages
LUNCH	Black Olive, Tomato and Onion Tart, Green Salad
DINNER	Lamb Chops with Cumin Minted Peas, Cauliflower Baked Potato with Sour Cream Lemon Sorbet

BREAKFAST	Porridge and Brown Sugar Milk or Cream
LUNCH	Sardine Salad with Radish, Cucumber, Onion
DINNER	Lasagna with Meat and Tomato Sauce, Grated Cheese Green Salad, Vinegar and Oil Fresh Fruit Salad

BREAKFAST	Smoked Haddock Sliced Oranges and Cream
LUNCH	Clear Consommé with Noodles Beef in Red Wine Braised Vegetable Platter Cheese Board with Celery Sticks
DINNER	Chive Omelet French Bread and Butter Apples and Nuts

SECOND WEEK

BREAKFAST	Crunchy Breakfast Cereal Milk or Cream
LUNCH	Raw Vegetable Platter Cheese and Onion Dip
DINNER	Stuffed Cabbage with Paprika Green Beans Celery and Walnut Salad Cheese Board

BREAKFAST	Scrambled Eggs and Bacon Toast and Preserves
LUNCH	Fresh Green Pea Soup with Diced Ham
DINNER	Fish Fillets with Almond Flakes Leeks in Cream Sauce Potato Straws Red Cabbage Salad Chocolate Mousse

BREAKFAST	Fried Eggs and Bacon Toast and Jam or Marmalade
LUNCH	Quick Cheese Souffle Green Salad, French Dressing
DINNER	Roast Lamb with Parsley Sauce Peas, Baby Turnips Roast Potatoes Vanilla Pudding with Fruit Sauce

BREAKFAST	Apple Pancakes with Sugar and Lemon Juice
LUNCH	Tomato Soup Maryland Fried Chicken Sauté Bananas, Corn Fritters Leaf Spinach, Green Salad and Cream
DINNER	White Beans and Brown Rice Salad Grated Carrot and French Dressing Orange Sherbert

High Fiber Diet

BULK AND BRAN

Fiber, the part of whole grains, fruits and vegetables that is not digestible (the bran in whole wheat or the cellulose in raw fruits and vegetables) is removed in the processing of much of our food. Five years ago you would not have even heard the word fiber mentioned in connection with nutrition. It was considered unnecessary simply because, unlike vitamins and minerals, fats, proteins and carbohydrates, it is not absorbed into the system. Nutritionists dismissed it as being superfluous to human needs.

No longer. Now many scientists believe that a lack of fiber in the modern Western diet is responsible for the rising level of a number of illnesses. It is lost in the refining of flour to make white bread, and the similar processing of sugar beets and cane to make white sugar.

Studies of people throughout the third world who live on diets of unrefined foods have turned up some fascinating evidence. Research showed that many of our common degenerative diseases – obesity, varicose veins, peptic ulcers, atherosclerosis, diabetes and dental problems – are practically unknown among these societies. At first, the conclusion was that there was some kind of natural immunity that protected them. These theories were proved wrong when immunity rapidly disappeared in the coastal regions where European and American residents and food manufacturers distributed over-refined and processed foods. The degenerative disease rate began to rise rapidly and the local population began to develop our Western illnesses.

The single most striking difference between the unrefined diets and our own is that in our diet the fiber had been removed.

It is not quite clear why the fiber should affect so many parts of the system. But one group of diseases linked to digestion and elimation are very responsive to additional bulk. A person eating unrefined foods has a very short 'transit time' of perhaps a few hours. This is the time it takes from putting food in the mouth until all the wastes are eliminated by the bowels. The transit time of refined food can be as much as a few days. This means that he can be unknowingly suffering from constipation even though he has a bowel movement every day and that all the wastes are probably not being eliminated rapidly enough from the body – a fact which many researchers also link with the increasing incidence of cancer of the bowel.

For these reasons, many doctors now recommend we all change to what is called a 'high fiber diet', eating as little as possible of sugar, white bread, pasta and other products made from white flour. Instead, we should be eating whole grains, fresh fruits and vegetables, lean meat, fish, fowl, and dairy products. Sound familiar? We've said it before! Additionally, such foods may offer other protective substances perhaps, as yet, unknown to nutritional science which might also prove to be helpful to the preservation of human health.

Additional bran can be a great boon to any regime for losing weight. Limited amounts of food, or too many protein foods, can often lead to constipation, but a few spoonfuls of bran a day will solve that. It is also good for providing bulk so that you don't feel so hungry. Try taking a couple of teaspoons or tablespoons half an hour before each meal with a glass of water. It will make you feel fuller when you sit down to eat so you are inclined to eat less.

Slimming research shows that bran in the intestines may actually decrease the amount of calories absorbed from other foods, and of course, you need not worry about any calories from the bran itself, as it is not absorbed but simply passes through the body.

Bran (which we have been discarding to keep as pig feed for the past century) is an excellent source of natural fiber and it is easy to buy and inexpensive to add to family dishes. But please don't imagine that bran alone is the answer to everything.

Obviously adding bran to a refined diet by sprinkling it on cereals or putting it into white bread and bakery goods is certainly better than eating an over-refined diet on its own. It will solve most constipation problems. But it doesn't make sense to think that you can continue to eat the same poor diet, simply add bran and get all the other health preserving benefits.

ADDING BRAN TO YOUR DIET

If you want to supplement your diet with bran, begin by taking one heaped teaspoon of bran three times a day. It can be washed down with juice or water, sprinkled on packaged breakfast cereals, mixed into porridge or added to soup. At first taking bran may blow up your stomach, or give you a gassy feeling but this will pass in a couple of weeks and won't recur. After two weeks gradually increase the amount of bran until *without straining*, your bowels move easily once, or better yet, twice a day. The amount of bran you will need varies a lot from person to person (usually between 3 teaspoons and 3 tablespoons a day). If you get lots of fresh fruit and vegetables you will need less. If you switch to wholegrain cereal products as well and avoid sugar and foods with sugar added you will probably not need it at all.

When eating bran, it is wise also to step up the amounts of fluids you drink. Liquid plays an important part in the action of the bran itself on the bowels. Try to drink six or eight glasses of liquid a day.

Make the change gradually, adding bran to baked things and you will find the family probably won't notice the difference.

High Fiber Menus

FIRST WEEK		SECOND WEEK	
BREAKFAST	¹/₂ Grapefruit Whole Bran Cereal with Sliced Apples	**BREAKFAST**	Orange Juice Porridge with added Bran Brown Sugar and Skim Milk
LUNCH	Leeks Vinaigrette Grated Carrot Salad Granary Toast	**LUNCH**	Cottage Cheese and Fresh Fruit Salad Wholemeal Toast
DINNER	Parslied Ham Potato and Green Pepper Casserole Mixed Salad, French Dressing Apricot Fluff	**DINNER**	Lamb Chops, very lean Leaf Spinach, Baked Potato Green Salad, Tarragon Dressing Cooked Prunes and Cream

BREAKFAST	Oatmeal Porridge with added Bran and Honey	**BREAKFAST**	¹/₂ Grapefruit Mixed Cereal with Skim Milk
LUNCH	Scrambled Eggs and Herbs Wholewheat Toast	**LUNCH**	Rasin, Carrot and Nut Salad Brown Rice
DINNER	Meat Loaf and Fresh Onion Gravy, Cauliflower with Cheese- Bran Topping Tomato Salad Rhubarb and Ginger	**DINNER**	Oven-Baked Fish with Lemon Sauce Potato and Celery Casserole Stuffed Tomatoes Cucumber and Olive Salad Cheese Board

BREAKFAST	Orange Juice Boiled Eggs and Toast Fingers	**BREAKFAST**	Poached Eggs on Toast Fruit Juice
LUNCH	Cheese Salad with Lettuce and Tomato Brown Bread	**LUNCH**	Home-made Paté with Crusty Bread, Pickles
DINNER	Chicken and Mushrooms on Brown Rice Green Peas in their Pods Red Cabbage Slaw Poached Whole Pears (with skins)	**DINNER**	Crisp Fried Chicken Barley and Mushroom Casserole Broccoli with Lemon Sauce Mixed Salad ¹/₂ Melon

FIRST WEEK		SECOND WEEK	
BREAKFAST	Fruit Juice Mixed Cereal with Skim Milk	**BREAKFAST**	Mushrooms on Brown Toast Sliced Oranges and Cream
LUNCH	Chicken Mayonnaise Red Apple Salad	**LUNCH**	Cheese and Ham Tart Green Salad
DINNER	Watercress Soup Veal Cutlet in Wine Brussels Sprouts Julienne Carrots Sauté Potatoes Cheese Board and Fruit	**DINNER**	Beef Stew (added Bran) Crisp-fried Cabbage Baked Potato Mixed Salad and Dressing Poached Dried Fruit Salad
BREAKFAST	1/2 Grapefruit Porridge and Sliced Bananas	**BREAKFAST**	All-Bran Cereal and Raisins Milk or Cream
LUNCH	Cottage Cheese with Sunflower Seeds Diced Fresh Fruit	**LUNCH**	Fresh Asparagus Soup Cheese and Crackers
DINNER	Baked Cod, Fresh Tomato Sauce Corn on the Cob Brussels Sprouts Plum Nut Pudding, Rum Topping	**DINNER**	Raw Vegetable Platter with Herb Sauces for Dipping Hot Apple Pudding
BREAKFAST	Bacon, Tomato and Sausage Wholemeal Toast	**BREAKFAST**	Oatmeal Porridge and Prunes Sliced Oranges
LUNCH	Lentil and Mushroom Soup Crusty Rolls	**LUNCH**	High Protein Spaghetti Butter and Grated Cheese
DINNER	Braised Ham with Peaches Creamed Potatoes Leaf Spinach, Green Salad Blackberry Crumble	**DINNER**	Ham and Mushroom Soufflé Green Salad, French Dressing Berries and Cream
BREAKFAST	Special K Cereal with Grated Apples, Milk	**BREAKFAST**	Hot Cereal, Stewed Prunes with added Bran
LUNCH	Artichoke Vinaigrette Roast Beef and Fresh Mushrooms Glazed Onions, Carrots Baked Parsnips and Potatoes Green Figs and Cream	**LUNCH**	Consommé with Noodles Roast Turkey with Stuffing Brussels Sprouts and Chestnuts Cranberry Sauce Garlic Green Salad Cheesecake
DINNER	Mixed Bean Salad Brown Rice Pilaf Cheese Board	**DINNER**	Grilled Bacon Sandwich Sliced Tomato Salad Apples and Nuts

Living Without Meat

A DIFFERENT WAY OF LIFE

Far from being a modern fad, vegetarianism is a well established way of living. Whole civilisations in the Far East and Asia have thrived on a meatless diet for thousands of years. Recently it has become a popular nutritional alternative in the West. Why do people become vegetarians? Some of the reasons for choosing a vegetarian diet are:

- Lower in fat, especially saturated fats often linked with heart disease
- Generally lower in calories (a high calorie diet is implicated in premature aging and degenerative diseases)
- Can be less costly than a conventional diet
- Ecologically sound
- Avoids chemicals used on animal farms and drugs such as hormone boosters which are added to animal feeds.

There's always a good reason for economy, especially with a large family to feed, and well planned meals of fresh fruits and vegetables, can be cheaper than a conventional diet that includes meat and expensive foods.

Some choose vegetarianism for philosophical or religious reasons, especially because of the protest against animal slaughter. Then there's ecology; animals raised on good agricultural land eat ten times the amount of food that we get from them as meat. Growing crops for direct human consumption would help stem the hunger in many countries in the world. Finally for health reasons; vegetarians on average consume less calories, significantly less fat and more roughage, two factors now linked with heart and other degenerative diseases. A sugarless vegetarian diet has also been tested for arthritis sufferers because it is less acid, and acids help in the elimination of toxins which contribute to the illness.

Becoming a vegetarian doesn't mean just giving up meat. It also means a change of attitude towards food, how it is made and eaten. A meatless diet of white bread, white sugar, overcooked vegetables and processed foods is even worse for you than the same diet with meat. At least the meat provides protein, vitamin D, and other nutrients.

One of the commonest beliefs is that meat is necessary for good health because it offers better quality protein than anything else. Not true; plants are perfectly capable of supplying all the protein, fat and carbohydrates essential for nutrition.

Just how nutritious a vegetarian diet is depends, just the same as any kind of diet, on who is planning it. Vegetables, fruits, nuts, grains and pulses are the best sources of minerals like calcium and magnesium, vitamin A, vitamin C, and E and the B complex group. Dairy products supply vitamin D. When you mix together pulses or legumes such as lentils or beans with cereal grains such as wheat, rice or corn, you get an excellent balance of the essential amino acids.

One of the medical professions' main objections to a vegetarian way of eating has been that a diet without meat or fish might mean a deficiency of vitamin B12 or to a far less degree vitamin D. B12 is most richly found in liver. It also occurs in kidney, muscle meat, fish, milk, eggs and cheese. It is an important vitamin for the health of the nervous system. A lack of it can lead to pernicious anaemia and nerve damage.

Vegetarians can take a supplement of B12 just to be absolutely sure they are getting enough but, provided their day to day diet includes a good quantity of milk, eggs and cheese, nutritionists now believe there is little danger.

MAKING VEGETARIANISM WORK

Before you experiment with a vegetarian diet, you should become familiar with a few basic principles. First you need to understand the question of protein and how to insure you are getting enough of the right kind. There are 22 amino acids, the building blocks of proteins, which are necessary for growth, health and reproduction. All but eight of these can be made in the body from others. These eight (Isoleucine, Leucine, Lysine, Methionine, Phenylalanine, Threonine, Tryptophan and Valine), usually called the essential amino acids, have to be supplied in the diet to be usable by the body in building its own proteins. They need to be eaten together at the same meal.

Meat and fish contain all these essential amino acids in a good balance which is why they are often called 'good quality' or 'complete' proteins. So do soya, acorns, cheese and eggs. Other foods such as nuts, grains (wheat, rye, corn, rice) and legumes

(red beans, lentils, dried beans) contain *most* of these essentials but are deficient in one or two. Eaten on their own, they won't supply all the body needs for health. So a vegetarian either replaces meat in the menu with soya, cheese or eggs or he chooses to mix together a grain with one of the legumes (brown rice with lentils) so that the deficient amino acids in one type of food will be made up in the other. This mixture will provide a very inexpensive, complete protein at any meal.

Nuts are also a rich source of protein. A mixture of brazil nuts, hazel nuts, cashews and sunflower seeds can be ground in a coffee grinder or a blender, and then stored in the refrigerator to make nut rissoles, or a loaf, or simply to sprinkle on vegetable dishes and salad. (Brazils are a good source of methionine, and sunflower seeds and cashews are high in lysine). The mixture not only supplies excellent quality protein, it is also rich in unsaturated fatty acids, important for the health of the circulation system, skin and brain cells.

Also, try to eat *half* of your foods raw. Fruits, vegetables cut into salads, nuts and sprouted seeds and grains offer the highest levels of naturally balanced vitamins, minerals and enzymes of any available foods. Along with whole grains, they are an excellent source of bulk. A salad, far from being a boring bowl of limp green, can become a good protein source, *and* the delicious focal point of a meal, when it is made of a variety of raw vegetables, then sprinkled with nuts, grated cheese, sunflower seeds or sprouted seeds, and grains for protein.

Vegetarian Menus

Family		Vegetarian	
BREAKFAST	Sliced Fresh Fruit with Flaked Bran and Cream	**BREAKFAST**	Sliced Fresh Fruit Flaked Bran and Cream
LUNCH	Chicken Salad Mayonnaise Green Pepper Salad	**LUNCH**	Celery and Walnut Salad Diced Green Peppers
DINNER	Baked Noodles and Cottage Cheese Green Salad, French Dressing Redcurrent Pudding	**DINNER**	Baked Noodle and Cottage Cheese Green Salad, French Dressing Redcurrant Pudding

BREAKFAST	¹/₂ Grapefruit Sausage and Tomato	**BREAKFAST**	¹/₂ Grapefruit Tomato and Fried Egg
LUNCH	Mushroom and Barley Soup Granary Bread	**LUNCH**	Mushroom and Barley Soup Granary Bread
DINNER	Fish Pie with Potato Topping Broccoli Corn and Red Peppers ¹/₂ Melon (Honeydew or Cantaloupe)	**DINNER**	Potato Topping only Broccoli with Melted Cheese Corn and Red Pepper Salad ¹/₂ Melon

BREAKFAST	Kippered Herring Fillets Wholewheat Toast	**BREAKFAST**	Muesli and Grated Apple Milk or Cream
LUNCH	Stuffed Eggs with Mustard Green Salad	**LUNCH**	Devilled Eggs with Mustard Green Salad
DINNER	Liver and Onions Fried Potatoes Cucumber and Radish Salad Fresh Fruit Salad with Coconut	**DINNER**	Beans Baked in Tomato Sauce Fried Potatoes Leaf Spinach with Cheese Cucumber and Radish Salad Fresh Fruit Salad and Coconut

Family		Vegetarian	
BREAKFAST	Crunchy Breakfast Cereal Milk or Cream	**BREAKFAST**	Crunchy Breakfast Cereal Milk or Cream Sliced Oranges
LUNCH	Raw Vegetable Platter Cheese and Onion Dip	**LUNCH**	Raw Vegetable Platter Cheese and Onion Dip
DINNER	Stuffed Cabbage with Paprika Green Beans Celery and Walnut Salad Cheese Board	**DINNER**	Stuffed Cabbage made with Rice only, no meat Green Beans Celery and Walnut Salad Cheese Board

Family		Vegetarian	
BREAKFAST	Scrambled Eggs and Bacon Toast and Preserves	**BREAKFAST**	Scrambled Eggs with Herbs Toast and Preserves
LUNCH	Fresh Green Pea Soup with Diced Ham	**LUNCH**	Fresh Green Pea Soup without Ham
DINNER	Fish Fillets with Almond Flakes Leeks in Cream Sauce Potato Straws Red Cabbage Salad Chocolate Mousse	**DINNER**	Leeks in Cream and Cheese Sauce Potato Straws Red Cabbage and Chestnuts Green Salad Chocolate Mousse

Family		Vegetarian	
BREAKFAST	Fried Eggs and Bacon Toast and Jam or Marmalade	**BREAKFAST**	Fruit Juice Tomato and Mushrooms
LUNCH	Quick Cheese Souffle Green Salad, French Dressing	**LUNCH**	Quick Cheese Soufflé with Diced Green Pepper Green Salad, French Dressing
DINNER	Roast Lamb with Parsley Sauce Peas, Baby Turnips Roast Potatoes Vanilla Pudding with Fruit Sauce	**DINNER**	Peas, Baby Turnips Barley Baked with Herbs Roast Potatoes Hard Cheese Vanilla Pudding with Fruit Sauce

Family		Vegetarian	
BREAKFAST	Apple Pancakes with Sugar and Lemon Juice	**BREAKFAST**	Apple Pancakes with Sugar and Lemon Juice
LUNCH	Tomato Soup Maryland Fried Chicken Sauté Bananas, Corn Fritters Leaf Spinach, Green Salad and Cream	**LUNCH**	Tomato Soup Baked Rice and Coconut Sauté Bananas, Corn Fritters Leaf Spinach, Green Salad Berries and Cream
DINNER	White Beans and Brown Rice Salad Grated Carrot and French Dressing Orange Sherbert	**DINNER**	White Bean and Brown Rice Salad Grated Carrot and French Dressing Orange Sherbert

73

Alternative Diets

THE VEGAN DIET

Vegans are vegetarians who shun dairy products such as milk, cheese, yogurt, cream and eggs as well as fish, fowl and meat. The Charter of the Vegan Society says 'Veganism is a way of living which excludes all forms of and cruelty to, the animal kingdom and includes a reverence and compassion for all life'.

The diet consists entirely of vegetables, fruits, nuts, grains and legumes. Vegans use soya plant food instead of milk, sweet agars instead of gelatine and soya flour or arrowroot for their sauces and gravies. Provided it follows the principles of a good vegetarian diet a vegan diet is capable of supporting an excellent level of health except for two things: it does not supply enough vitamin B12 nor enough vitamin D.

Vitamin D can be obtained from sunlight, and it is also often added to margarines, which vegans eat. But B12 is a different matter. With the exception of traces which occur in wheat germ, brewer's yeast, soya, and the herb comfrey, vitamin B12, which is necessary for the health of the blood and nervous system, is not found in vegetable foods. It is made in the intestines of animals and stored in the liver. And although there are thousands of perfectly healthy vegan children in the world who have never been given supplements, a meat eater whose body has been used to a normal level of B12, and who switches to a vegan diet, is likely to suffer deficiencies after the body's store is used up. This is why many vegans take B12, in a supplement, as well as added to plant milk made from soya beans.

MACROBIOTICS

Organic grains, vegetables, seeds and a little home-grown fruit form the basis of the macrobiotic diet.

It is based on the highly metaphysical classification of foods into 'yin' and 'yang' and the macrobiotic diet is an attempt to achieve the perfect balance between the two. Yin and yang are not just food groups, they are part of a well developed Eastern philosophy of life that has been applied to every human need, including medicine, exercise, social relationships and art. Yin is said to have the qualities of cold, dark, passivity, vegetable, and it is basically feminine. Yang is supposed to be light, heat, activity and masculine. The yin foods include mainly vegetables and fruits; sugar comes way down the list. Yang foods are meat, fish and salty things. Cooked cereals, particularly whole brown rice, lie between the two and therefore are said to be balanced. Macrobiotic followers avoid sugar in any form, all food additives, and rarely touch meat or fish. The ideal diet is said to be one of pure grains (usually plain brown rice) with a little cooked vegetables and seeds. Doctors and nutritionists warn it can lead to serious vitamin and mineral deficiencies. Certainly a macrobiotic diet requires deep understanding of the philosophy and a complete re-education of cooking habits to be successful.

FOOD COMBINING:
DON'T MIX FOODS THAT FIGHT

It's not only what and how much you eat, but what you eat with what. That is the principle behind careful food combining. It was once known as the Hay diet, named for the doctor who's one simple commandment was 'don't mix proteins or acid fruits with carbohydrates at the same meal'.

It may sound strange, but there are a great many people who believe that following such a diet has had a positive effect on their digestive problems. We do know that concentrated proteins such as meat, fish, poultry, eggs and cheese need an acid medium for complete digestion, while carbohydrates (sugars and starches) need an alkaline medium. If both are in the digestive system together, the enzymes which break down the foods conflict with each other, and cannot do their work as thoroughly as they should. This is especially true in older people, whose systems may not be too efficient.

The simplest practical menu is to eat one protein, one starch and one alkaline meal each day, so you keep the foods separate, but you get enough of each group for good health.

Protein Meals
Fresh meats, fish, game, poultry, eggs, cheese, nuts.
Eat only with:
Acid fruits, such as apples, apricots, cherries, grapefruit, nectarines, berries, prunes.
Vegetables such as green and root vegetables (except potatoes).

Salads: cabbage, celery, cress, lettuce, tomatoes, peppers.

Starch Meals
Cereals, meusli, oatmeal, brown rice, breads, pasta, cakes, all made where possible from wholemeal flours, without eggs.
Eat only with:
Sugars, though not too much, made from honey, dates, figs, ripe bananas, etc.
Vegetables such as any green or root vegetable, including potatoes.
Salads as listed above, except for tomatoes – cooked only.

Alkaline Meals
Yogurt or Milk (unsweetened).
Eat only with:
Any green or root vegetable, any acid fruit (see Protein meal for list).

Not recommended at any time:
Dried peas or beans, chestnuts, rhubarb, vinegar, pickles, hot spices, foods containing much sugar.

Low Blood Sugar

LOW BLOOD SUGAR

Do you find yourself strangely depressed for no real reason, as well as feeling tired almost all the time? Drinking endless cups of coffee doesn't help, it gives you a lift for a little while, but then you feel let down all over again. If you seem to want sweet things all the time, too, then perhaps you might benefit from a diet designed to avoid low blood sugar.

Low blood sugar is a condition with different and very varied symptoms, and there are some doctors who believe it doesn't even exist. On balance, there are quite a few diet experts who feel that low blood sugar lies behind a number of common ailments – general physical weakness, migraine and back pain, alcohol addiction and depression. They say it is particularly common among crash dieters, housewives and young mothers, – all those who don't take the trouble to eat well-balanced meals day after day.

Briefly, this is what it is all about; the tissues of the brain, the nerves and the red-blood cells depend on a small but constant supply of sugar, which is converted into energy to help them work well. Eating a little sugar now and then, as happens in a normal diet, is enough to keep the energy level just right. However, if it's a long time between meals, or there is a temporary block in the glucose-supplying mechanism, you may react by feeling nervous, faint and slightly irritable. Even eating a light snack – an apple or a piece of cheese – is enough to bring the blood sugar level back to normal, and the symptoms disappear.

It would seem that having the right level is profoundly important to your general health and emotional balance, and the wrong level can alter your moods and your physical state in a way we don't quite understand.

We do know that the pancreas controls the sugar level by secreting insulin. When there is too little insulin in the blood-stream, it can't control the sugar properly, the level goes way up, and diabetes develops. But when the pancreas makes too *much* insulin all the time, it keeps the level too low, and the tissues that depend on that sugar are starved of energy.

There are many reasons why the pancreas over-secretes insulin. Strangely, one of the major causes is continually eating too much sugar. Large quantities of refined sugar overstimulate the pancreas, making it trigger happy so it produces too much insulin, too often. The insulin produced in turn pushes blood sugar levels even lower. You feel tired, crave food (particularly sweet and starchy food). Yet taking in more sugar only worsens the situation in a kind of unhappy circle. A pattern many chronic dieters know only too well!

But for a problem that can cause untold miseries, low blood sugar can be surprisingly simple to treat. You need only make a few changes in your diet. First, stop eating sugar (and this means chocolates, cola drinks, and sweet cakes as well as the sugar that goes on grapefruit and in coffee.) It is easy to get all the energy you need from natural sugar in other foods in your diet. And avoid the concentrated sweetness of refined sugar – it is too strong a stimulus to the pancreas. So are coffee and cola drinks, so drink one of the coffee substitutes or decaffinated coffee instead. Eat a good variety of natural foods (the precooked, processed foods often have hidden sugar), including plenty of protein. Finally, eat something like a piece of cheese every two hours throughout the day. This usually is enough to keep the blood-sugar at the right level so unpleasant symptoms don't develop.

One point, though – the symptoms of low blood sugar are very much like the symptoms of other physical and mental problems – anaemia, for example, can also make you feel tired, depressed and so on. So check with your doctor to make sure the cause isn't something else which needs medical treatment.

Research shows that low-blood-sugar is most common among women. Too many housewives skimp on the quality of the food they eat themselves although they make sure their families are well fed. Many women, without realizing it, exist on a diet of coffee and carbohydrates. If you happen to be one of them, there is only one way to find out what an anti-low-blood-sugar diet could do for you; try it.

FOODS TO ELIMINATE

Ale

Beer

Wine

Cocktails

Coffee (unless decaffinated)

Strong tea

Very cold drinks

Soft drinks sweetened with sugar such as colas and sweetened fruit juices

Chocolate, cocoa

Canned fruit in syrup

Sugar, honey, candy, cakes, tarts, pies, puddings, ice cream, pastries

Fruits that are high in sugar content such as raisins, dates, figs, plums, bananas, grapes

Large quantities of pasta and white bread

FOODS TO EAT

Proteins: Meat, fish, poultry, eggs, milk, nuts, cheese.

Vegetables: All green leafy vegetables plus broccoli, avocados, brussel sprouts, celery, cucumbers, corn, cauliflower, tomatoes, squash, turnips, peas, onions, radishes, beans and artichokes.

Fruits: Grapefruit, oranges, lemons, tangerines, all berries, pears, apples, melons.

Drinks: Decaffinated coffee, weak tea, herb teas, coffee substitutes (all sweetened with artificial sweeteners only), distilled liquors, natural fruit juices.

Low Blood Sugar Menus

Since the variations on this diet are limited, we have listed only the recommended changes. Keep to all the usual guides for good nutrition.

FAMILY

DIETER

BREAKFAST	Oatmeal Porridge Cream Toast and Preserves	**BREAKFAST**	No Toast unless special high protein bread Add bran where possible to dishes
LUNCH	Grapefruit and Cottage Cheese Salad	**DINNER**	No added bread or cereal to burgers – use pure meat, or eggs for binding
DINNER	Clear Soup with Parsley Spicy Pork and Veal Burgers Split Rolls Tomato Halves Cheese and Fruit		Serve without rolls Choose apple or pear

BREAKFAST	¹/₂ Grapefruit Scrambled Eggs and Bacon Toast	**LUNCH**	No potato salad Add extra coleslaw plus sliced tomato
LUNCH	Cold Meat Platter Potato Salad Coleslaw	**DINNER**	Small baked potato is allowed
DINNER	Fried Liver and Onions Leaf Spinach Baked Potatoes Caramel Custard		

BREAKFAST	Sliced Oranges and Bananas Cream	**BREAKFAST** **DINNER**	Sliced oranges only Use High-Protein or Soy Flour Lasagna – make one section with extra meat sauce
LUNCH **DINNER**	Tuna Fish salad with Anchovies Lasagna Romana made with meat Green Salad Apples and Cheese board		

FAMILY

BREAKFAST	Orange Juice Egg and Sausage Toast
LUNCH	Mixed Grill (liver, tomatoes, sausage) Fried Egg
DINNER	Lamb, and Green Pepper Kebabs Plain Rice Pilaf Mixed Salad Yoghurt Sauce Mint Chiffon Dessert

BREAKFAST	Muesli and Yoghurt Grated Apple
LUNCH	Cream of Chicken Soup Crusty French Bread
DINNER	Baked Hungarian Fish Braised Red Cabbage Sauté Potatoes Pineapple Cheesecake

BREAKFAST	Orange Juice Smoked Haddock Toast
LUNCH	Raw Spinach and Bacon Salad
DINNER	Russian Egg Salad Roast Chicken with Pork and Onion Stuffing Baked Potatoes Strawberry Parfait

BREAKFAST	Melon Cup Fresh Rolls
LUNCH	Farmhouse Beef Casserole Green Beans Mixed Garlicky salad Baked Gingered Apple
DINNER	Chicken pancakes

DIETER

DINNER	No rice Serve extra kebab Dessert made with plain gelatin and artificial sweetener

BREAKFAST	No muesli Extra grated apple and plain unsweetened yoghurt
LUNCH	No bread Soup made without flour – use egg or cream to thicken Add diced meat
DINNER	No potatoes Extra fish (for Saturday) Cake served without crust

LUNCH	Piece of cold fish from Friday night
DINNER	Stuffing made with pure meat, no cereals or bread used No potato

BREAKFAST	Make boiled or poached egg
DINNER	Serve creamed chicken filling as omelet without pancakes

79

10-80-10 Diet

LIVING LONGER

As a result of increasing evidence of links between what we eat and the illnesses we suffer from, nutrition has become a tool of preventive medicine. Research teams have been looking for specific guidelines to help us live longer, and slow down the frightening growth in degenerative diseases such as diabetes, coronary heart disease, gout and hypertension. One suggested guideline is known as the 10%–80%–10% diet, because it advocates taking 10% of your calories from protein foods, another 10% from fats and 80% from unrefined carbohydrates. It is little short of a revolution in the average person's eating habits.

Researchers have discovered some important differences between ourselves and rural communities who develop very few of our degenerative problems. Where almost half our calories come from fats, a bare 5 to 10% of their calories are taken in the form of fat or oil. We eat a lot of salt, they eat very little. We take in about 400 milligrams of caffeine a day in coffee; they take generally none at all. We consume large quantities of refined sugar, which is virtually unknown among primitive peoples. We are also big meat and egg eaters, both high in cholesterol.

From these observations, doctors have made a list of recommendations for a new way of life. They believe it will keep our bodies in good condition, and free of many chronic illnesses for as long as possible. The diet plus regular exercises was tried out on a number of people of different ages and with varying physical conditions from advanced diabetes and heart disease, to normal health.

The results seem to show that everyone in the scheme benefited, and the long life system was made available as an alternative to the normal balanced diet.

It sounds simple, but in practice, this means a considerable change in your eating habits: only 3 to 4 ounces of meat or fish a day, no added salt (there is enough natural salts in vegetables) and no dairy products (except non-fat ones). It also means you need to cut out sugar and all refined carbohydrates completely which includes everything from cereals containing sugar to honey, cakes and sweets. Finally, you must stop drinking coffee and tea and use herb teas instead.

If you decide to follow the 10%–80%–10% diet the change over to it should be gradual. First cut down on sugar and fats. Then increase your use of wholegrain cereals and dishes made from wheat, brown rice, corn and buckwheat and pulses plus vegetables and salads.

For most of us it is a very difficult and unsociable change to make – no restaurants, no visiting at friends' houses and complete avoidance of some of the most traditional and festive family meals. But there is no denying that remarkable improvements have been reported by people suffering from chronic illnesses. Undoubtedly the emphasis on regular exercise is part of the reason for success and that is something everyone should copy.

FOODS TO EAT

Wholegrain breads (without oil, shortening or salt added to recipe)

Wholegrain cereals like shredded wheat, wheat flakes, meusli (without sugar)

Wholegrain cooked cereals like rolled oats or wheat flakes

Crackers made without salt

Skimmed milk

Eggs (use the whites only)

Cheese – only defatted kinds

Fruit juices (without added sugar)

Fish (preferably sole, halibut and other low-fat varieties)

Chicken or Turkey (preferably white meat)

Meat (lean only, not marbled, no sausages of any kind, hamburgers, organ meats or sandwich meats)

Whole grains: brown rice, barley, buckwheat

Bean: soya, kidney, navy, lima etc

Onions and spices (but not pre-mixed varieties which contain additives)

Vegetables: All kinds

Fruits: (but avoid avocados, olives and nuts, no sweetened, processed fruit)

Pastas and noodles: (preferably the whole wheat varieties … avoid spinach noodles and other noodles containing eggs)

SIX BASIC PRINCIPLES

1. **Avoid Fat**
    This means eliminating butter, margarine and shortening in cooking; oily plants like avocado and nuts; dairy products (except non-fat dairy products); and fatty meats.

2. **Avoid Sugar**
    This means no pies, cakes, or pastries; no cereals containing sugar; no syrups, molasses or honey, nothing to which sugar has been added.

3. **Avoid Salt**
    Don't use it at the table or in your cooking. Eat no foods (such as crackers) which are salted.

4. **No Coffee or Tea**
    Drink herb teas or fruit juice instead.

5. **Little Meat and No Extra Cholesterol**
    Keep your meat or fish intake down to 3 or 4 ounces a day. Eat no shellfish, eggs, or animal organs such as liver, kidneys, or brains.

6. **Get Regular Exercise**

It's not really possible to include adaptable menus for the 10%–80%–10%, because basic cooking habits must change and family meals prepared in the ordinary way are just not practical.

Learn to read labels carefully. Many processed and frozen foods have sugar, eggs and fats added. Make all stews and soups in advance so you can skim off the fat when it has chilled, then re-heat.

Some useful substitutes:

Use skim milk instead of whole milk.

Use two egg whites instead of one whole egg.

Sugar substitutes: Puréed fruit such as apples, bananas, raisins, or concentrated (but *not* sweetened) frozen fruit juices.

A cream substitute: Blend skim milk cheese with a little skim milk until the right texture is achieved.

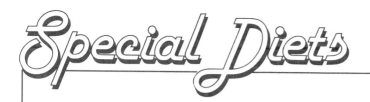

ALLERGIES

Most people think of allergies as something pretty straightforward – the running nose and red eyes of hay fever, sneezing when a cat comes into the room, coming out in spots after eating strawberries. These are certainly allergies, and very troublesome ones at that. But at least the cause and effect is easy to see, and you can avoid triggering off the reaction by simply keeping away from whatever it is that causes this irritation. But allergies don't always have such clear patterns, and doctors are becoming more and more careful about giving simple answers to complicated questions. There have been too many flat statements about the reason for many minor illnesses, and too little attention paid to individual reactions which vary enormously.

As information piles up, doctors have realized that all kinds of apparently unrelated symptoms can be caused by allergic reactions to foods, chemicals, and commonly used additives. Because our foods contain so many different elements, it can be very difficult to track down the culprit.

If you suffer from a recurring problem of any kind that doesn't seem to be caused by germs or infection, it may be an allergic reaction to something you eat. Sudden rashes, upset stomachs, vomiting and nausea, swollen fingers or ankles, headaches – all can be allergic reactions. Check with your doctor first.

Keep a record of everything you eat. A diary is a great help, because it is easy to fill it in every day. If the allergy is to something you eat often, then it should show up fairly quickly. For example, you may see in your diary that whenever the rash or other symptom appears, you had eaten eggs for breakfast.

Many people are allergic to quite basic foods; milk, eggs, cheese and wheat set off quite strong reactions. MSG an additive (monosodium-glutamate) causes an allergic reaction sometimes referred to as the Chinese Restaurant Syndrome which is characterized by shortness of breath, increased pulse rate, and headache. It usually goes away within an hour or two.

When you think you have spotted the cause, try leaving out one ingredient, or changing the cooking method. If you always react to strawberries and cream, it may be the strawberries, it may be the cream, or it may also be the chemical which that strawberry farmer used to spray his crop. Eggs and bacon may seem to trigger off a bad reaction, but it could be the eggs, the bacon, or the fat you use for frying. A little trial and error should help.

If you can't seem to find the answer, see your doctor. There are tests today for almost every kind of allergy, and vaccines are sometimes useful in controlling or limiting the effect.

ARTHRITIS

The damage caused by arthritis is stupendous. Three types have severe crippling effects and often grow progressively worse as the patient ages, adding even more pain and discomfort to the natural changes of growing old. Rheumatoid arthritis and ostioarthritis are the worst – literally millions of people suffer from their effect. Gout is also an arthritic disease, and it's always been accepted that gout is linked to certain foods which make it more or less painful. Since gout is a type of arthritis, it seemed possible that the other forms might also be responsive to certain foods in the diet.

As yet, there have not been sufficient studies to give a scientific answer, but a recommended diet based on fish, seafood, vegetables and rice has been devised by a doctor and seems to have had a positive effect on thousands of arthritis sufferers. Everyone has slightly different reactions, but it certainly worked for many previously crippled patients and it is worth trying if you have the disease.

In general, avoid all milk products, meat and chocolate. Shop carefully and read labels carefully for excessive additives and chemicals. Plan your diet primarily around fish and other seafood, vegetables, and rice. Avoid meat and poultry as much as possible.

ARTERIOSCLEROSIS

Arteriosclerosis, or hardening of the arteries, is a condition that results when the blood vessels become clogged with minerals and fatty materials and prevents the blood from flowing smoothly to all the cells of the body. Hardening of the arteries usually affects people over sixty, but it is a disease that develops slowly and therefore begins years before.

A number of signs indicate that arteriosclerosis has set in. There may be numbness or coldness in the extremeties, particularly the hands and feet. The thinking processes may be impaired with the memory becoming less acute. In later stages, the extremeties show signs of cramping, aching, or sharp pain. If the arteries to the brain are severely affected a stroke may result and can cause complete loss of memory and decreased control of normal body functions.

Arteriosclerosis is a very serious disease. If you suspect that you could have it or are showing signs that it might develop, consult your physician. With regard to diet, the doctor will probably limit the amount and type of fat you can consume. The consumption of eggs is usually cut considerably. Fish oils and vegetable oils do not contain saturated fatty acids which lead to high cholesterol levels in the blood, and therefore the doctor will probably recommend that you use only these and avoid all animal fats which have an abundance of this type of fatty material.

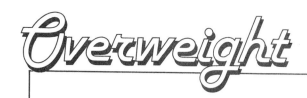

TAKING IT OFF

If you weigh 10 % more than you should, it can be detrimental to your health. 20 % more, and your weight becomes a serious medical complication. Yet about half of us in the West now weigh too much, and one in ten of us is severely overweight or obese. Overweight people die sooner and are more prone to disease of the cardio-vascular system, kidneys, liver and gall bladder than their lean friends. If you are overweight, you are also more accident prone and more likely to get diabetes and other degenerative illnesses, not to mention having to deal with the emotional pressure the heavy person has to cope with in our 'lean-oriented' society. That's all the bad news. The good news is that all of these hazards disappear when excess pounds are shed.

The primary causes of overweight are uncertain in spite of all the dogmatic statements that are made. No two people are alike. One individual's metabolism can burn up any amount of calories without putting an ounce of excess fat on the body. Another person eats very little, and it all seems to turn to fat. So metabolic differences between individuals have a lot to do with overweight. And serious disturbances can sometimes make you fat. But such problems are more likely to be the result of overweight than the cause of it. Childhood feeding patterns are an important factor too. If a child is overfed, or introduced to too many solid carbohydrate foods too early in life a larger number of fat cells than normal are laid down in his body. Later, he will have a greater tendency to get fat and stay that

way. And bottle-fed babies tend to be fatter when they grow up than breast-fed babies. Genetics can also play a part. A child with an overweight mother or father is more likely to become fat himself than an offspring of two lean parents.

If you want to be slim it probably matters what *kind* of diet you eat as well. Researchers studying different eating patterns throughout the world have repeatedly linked obesity with the widespread consumption of convenience foods and refined carbohydrates. This is probably because refined foods like white sugar and products made from white flour are highly concentrated sources of calories. They are too quickly and easily absorbed into the system. Try comparing how many slices of white bread you can *comfortably* eat with the same quantity of whole grain variety, although the calories in each are approximately the same.

Some people are lucky. They can get away with eating a lot of food without putting on weight. We still have no idea why this is so. If the doctors ever discover the answer, we will be a long way towards solving the fat problem.
In the meantime if you are overweight, it's better to face the fact that today, unfortunately, there are no secret formulas for slimming. Diet pills such as amphetamines, designed to curb your appetite are not the answer. Not only do they not work, they can seriously damage the body as a whole, greatly disturbing your emotional balance too. Special supplement formulas like taking vitamin B6, kelp and cider vinegar at each meal may be useful to some, but only as an

adjunct to a well designed weight loss regime. On their own they will do nothing.

If you are too fat, no amount of rationalizations about your metabolism is going to do anything about it. First you need to examine your mental attitude towards overweight and decide if you really want to lose those excess pounds. (Many people like worrying about their weight but unconsciously want to do little about changing it.) Once you are clear about what you want, you're ready to begin.

Successful dieting will come only through two things: appetite control plus a diet that supplies the body with less energy than it burns up through metabolism and activity day after day. Add an exercise program to improve your overall muscle and skin tone, and a relaxation technique to deal with stress that can turn to compulsive eating, and you are well on your way.

Which diet you choose depends on you, your lifestyle and personal preferences. For some, calorie counting is the best way. For others, an all-protein diet or carbohydrate-limited diet is better. Whichever you choose it is only a temporary means to an end. After your goal weight is achieved you should turn to a maintenance diet that fulfills all your long-term nutritional needs, and stay on it. For help with the appetite control, you can use some of the highly successful techniques of behavourists weight control (see next page). For any weight loss regime to work – that is, to take off pounds and *keep* them off – it should deal with four basic needs.

CHECK LIST FOR LOSING WEIGHT:

1. There should be no side effects, caused by drugs or vitamin or mineral deficiencies.

2. Re-educate your appetite for long lasting results.

3. Re-adjust the energy balance so you take in fewer calories than you burn up (this means diet and exercise).

4. You should try to change your attitude towards yourself, understanding what makes you eat plus an increased awareness of your emotional needs and how to fulfill them so you don't have to misuse food as a substitute for love or contentment.

CALORIES

Strictly speaking, a calorie is the amount of heat needed to raise the temperature of one gramme by one point centigrade.
In everyday language, we use calories to mean the amount of carbohydrate/starch in any one food which our bodies burn up for energy.
When we take in too many calories, the excess is stored as fat instead of being burned away.

Weight Control

THE HABIT OF LOSING WEIGHT

The habit-forming approach to losing weight is simple; regardless of built-in tendencies to gain weight, most excess poundage is the result of bad eating habits developed over many years. Why these habits develop is a complicated subject, and the reasons vary from person to person. Forget the background for the moment. Instead, deal with the results; too much fat. We may not find it easy to understand why we want to eat three portions of chocolate cake, but we can learn to control ourselves and eat something with less calories.

It doesn't demand great will power, yet the habit-control techniques can be effective in getting you slim and staying that way. Surprisingly, overweight people seldom have the pangs of real hunger that people of normal weight feel. They eat too much out of boredom, unconsciously nibble while watching television, or eat rapidly whatever food has been put on their plates.

This curious 'habit-eating' can be turned to advantage; become aware of exactly what habits are causing the trouble, and work to change bad habits to good ones. It's a question of self-education, that's all. It may sound too simple to be true, but such techniques are now successfully used to manage all kinds of problems from smoking to drug addiction. The following check chart approach provides the perfect tool for appetite control to go with any of the sensible weight loss diets given on the next pages. It is also something you can do yourself, without a lot of bolstering up. Forget

'I can't diet no matter how hard I try'. You can.

Before you begin any diet, use our weekly chart to note down when, where and how you eat (no matter how small a nibble or even a taste) and your feelings before and after each meal. It's important to be honest – this will make you aware of what habitually makes you want to eat. Perhaps you absent mindedly pick up a few nuts or a piece of fruit while you're on the telephone, especially if the bowl is too near, or every time you come into the house you automatically head for the refrigerator. These things don't happen by chance.

Learn to know what you do, then, using the basic steps we list, change your response, and if necessary your surroundings – move the fruit bowl, go into your bedroom instead of the kitchen, and so forth.
To begin with you will stop picking at bits of food that add up surprisingly quickly. Then with new habits and better planning any good diet will work. If you need added reminders, make a new check chart for yourself once a week, or once a month, to hold on to your new habits, and keep yourself slim and healthy.

Step One – Put everything on record
Keep track of your progress, your slip-ups, your difficulties, then you can take conscious steps to re-arrange external stimulus so you replace old negative habits with positive ones.
DECIDE TO RECORD YOUR EATING HABITS.
DECIDE TO RECORD YOUR EXERCISES.
DECIDE TO RECORD YOUR PERSONAL REACTIONS.

Step Two – Where do you eat?

It matters a lot. Overweight people are stimulated to eat by outside factors, the time on the clock, the sight of food, a feeling of loneliness. Limit the number of places you eat in and you'll limit your food intake.

DECIDE TO EAT IN ONLY ONE ROOM.
DECIDE TO EAT IN ONLY ONE PLACE IN THAT ROOM.
DECIDE TO DO NOTHING ELSE WHILE YOU'RE EATING.

Step Three – What do you eat?

Everyone has special temptation foods. Eliminate the fattening results by simply not keeping them in the house.

ELIMINATE TEMPTATION FOODS FROM YOUR SHOPPING LIST.

Step Four – How does your food look?

Research shows that the overweight person is strongly affected by visual contact with food. Served on a small plate he feels more satisfied than on a big one. When it is attractively presented it is also more satisfying.

DECIDE TO USE A SMALL PLATE.
DECIDE TO USE MEASURED QUANTITIES OF FOOD SO YOU KNOW HOW MUCH YOU ARE EATING.
DECIDE TO MAKE YOUR FOOD LOOK AS GOOD AS POSSIBLE.

Step Five – How fast do you eat?

Eat slowly and you'll eat less and feel more full.

DECIDE TO PUT YOUR FORK DOWN AFTER EACH BITE.
DECIDE TO CHEW EACH BITE TWENTY TIMES.
DECIDE TO TAKE NO MORE FOOD INTO YOUR MOUTH UNTIL WHAT IS ALREADY IN IT IS SWALLOWED.

Step Six – How do you keep your spirits up?

Many overweight people eat from boredom, fatigue or depression, making food compensate for other parts of their life they neglect.

DECIDE TO EAT REGULAR MEALS WITH A TIMETABLE.
DECIDE TO GET ENOUGH SLEEP AND RELAXATION.
DECIDE TO INCREASE YOUR PARTICIPATION IN ACTIVITIES NOT CONNECTED WITH FOOD.

Step Seven – The exercise factor

Exercise not only burns calories, it also raises your spirits and increases metabolic efficiency.

FIND AN EXERCISE OR SPORT YOU ENJOY, AND STICK TO IT.
DECIDE TO WALK BRISKLY AS MUCH AS YOU CAN EVERY DAY.

DAY OF THE WEEK	THE FOOD YOU EAT		
	WHAT YOU ATE AND HOW MUCH	WHEN	WHERE
MONDAY			
TUESDAY			
WEDNESDAY			
THURSDAY			
FRIDAY			
SATURDAY			
SUNDAY			

WITH WHOM	WHAT DID YOU FEEL LIKE BEFORE YOU ATE	WHAT DID YOU FEEL LIKE AFTER YOU ATE	WERE YOU DOING ANYTHING ELSE

Calorie Control Diet

COUNTING CALORIES

The most well known and commonly used form of weight control is counting calories. Its theory is simple: when energy output exceeds energy input, fat is reduced.

The average man of normal weight needs something between 2,500 and 3,000 calories a day, the average woman between 2,000–2,300. If we take in less than this, hormones and enzymes in the system which mobilise energy reserves from our fat cells will go into action, stored-up fat will be decreased, and we will gradually lose weight. *How* gradually depends on how few calories you take in daily.

It is fairly easy to work out. Each ounce of stored fat provides about 250 calories of energy so if you need 2,300 calories a day but are eating only 1,800 you will have a calorie deficit of 500 calories. This means you should lose about a pound a week. If you want to lose more you simply decrease the number of calories you are taking in each day.

Of course it is important to be sensible about this. It is useless to starve yourself so you have a calorie deficit of 1,500 a day if you are so hungry after a few days that you can't keep it up, and you jeopardize the whole diet by eating everything in sight.

There are nutritional considerations that are important too. You still have the same vitamins, minerals, protein, carbohydrate and fat requirements as non-slimmers. It is important to take them into consideration

and to do some careful menu planning otherwise you can end up with a slim waistline but an awful disposition, bad skin, or worse – serious illness.

In any calorie controlled diet you need to be sure to get plenty of green leafy vegetables (easy as they are very low in calories) in the form of salads. Make one meal a day a big salad from a variety of raw vegetables such as carrots, tomatoes, lettuce, cabbage, mushrooms, cucumber, celery green and red peppers and so forth. Learn to make low calorie salad dressings to add variety. It will go a long way towards fulfilling your vitamin and mineral needs.

You should also have one or two pieces of fruit a day, a good helping of lean protein food such as meat, fish, low fat cheese, or poultry and 2 slices of wholegrain bread, for bulk and the valuable B complex vitamins it contains. These are particularly important when dieting for maintaining high energy levels and counteracting the diet depression that leads to binges of fattening foods.

Liver, also a rich source of vitamins from the B group, is an excellent food for dieters. It is good to prepare it a couple of times a week if possible. If you suffer from constipation add three teaspoons of bran a day to your foods. Beyond this you can choose to use up your calorie allowance as you please, even indulging in a piece of chocolate a day as a reward if you need to.

Buy yourself a little calorie counter that lists all the energy values for the foods you eat and keep track each day of how much of your daily allowance is used up at each meal. You will have to measure and weigh your foods carefully to begin with until you become familiar with portion sizes and calorie values. Then staying within your limits and making calculations will become almost second nature.

To help you decide what is a good calorie limit for your weight loss, consider just how much you want to lose, then how physically active you are and how accustomed you are to eating fairly large meals. If you are a large eater, quite active and even if you want to lose more than 25 pounds then it is best to try for no less than 1,500 calories a day. If you do not eat much at one meal, have less weight to lose and are not terribly active physically, you will probably be able to manage on 1,000 calories.

If you are self disciplined, and do not use up too much energy, plan your Monday to Friday intake for 800 calories, then of Saturday and Sunday you will have 1,300 calories each day to fit your diet more easily into your family life.

You may find taking your food in several small snacks instead of three meals a day is a more satisfying way of eating, and there is some evidence to show it helps to speed food through your digestive system.

The key to success is perserverance. Results that come after weeks of calorie restrictions are more likely to be lasting than the quick weight loss from crash diets.

BASIC PRINCIPLES

1. Set yourself a daily (or weekly) calorie allowance and keep to it. Be sure to record everything you eat and drink in a notebook and add up the calories they contain. Weigh foods at first for careful calculation.

2. Stick to regular meal patterns, eating from 3 to 5 times a day and make your lightest meal dinner, if possible.

3. Include one portion of high protein food like meat, fish, poultry, or low fat cheese in your daily calorie allowance.

4. Eat lots of green vegetables, preferably raw, in mixed salads with low calorie dressings. Chew crisp, raw celery, cucumber or carrots when you're hungry between meals.

5. Eat 2 slices of wholegrain bread a day.

6. Don't add fat to foods unnecessarily. Bake or poach instead of frying.

7. Avoid alcohol as much as you can, except for an occasional glass of dry white wine.

8. Steer clear of all high calorie starchy foods like biscuits, cakes, pastry and sweets. They are empty foods without any real nutritional value. Look for low calorie alternatives to everything.

9. Take bran if you suffer from constipation.

10. Weigh yourself every week and record the results in your notebook at the same time. After getting up, and before you get dressed is the most encouraging.

Calorie Check Calorie

CALORIE COUNTING – A CONCISE CHART TO GET YOU STARTED

Counting calories can be difficult to judge unless you are careful to weigh all your portions, and check them against a detailed calorie chart. For most of us, though, it is enough to understand something about how the different foods measure up in an average calorie count. Remember that these are listed by portion, in order to make it easier for you to count your calories quickly and easily, but portions and sizes vary so much it is really impossible to give accurate measures – a 'small' apple can be 3 oz, 4 oz, or 5 oz, depending on the type and season.

A green apple contains less sugar than a ripe one, too. If you want to be more precise, then buy a pamphlet or paperback book which lists all the calorie values, by ounce, and buy an accurate pair of scales. Make sure your book includes manufactured foods; they vary quite a lot from one brand to another.

Almonds, 15 shelled	150
Ground, 1 tsp	10
All-bran, 1 bowl	160
Anchovies, 3 whole	18
Apple Cider, dry, per glass	115
Sweet cider	150
Apple Pie, 1 wedge	240
Apples, raw, 1 small	45
1 large	85
1 large cooking	100
1 baked, with sugar	180
Apple sauce, 1 tblsp	25
Apricots, raw, 3 small	50
in syrup, 6 halves	150
dried, per half	18

Artichoke, globe 1 whole large	25
with vinaigrette sauce	100
Jerusalem, boiled	15
Asparagus, per spear	4
Soup, 1 bowl	120
Avocado, half	170
with vinaigrette sauce	250
Bacon, 2 small slices	70
Fried	100
Bamboo shoots, fresh	25
Bananas, 1 whole small	75
1 large	100
Barley, pearl, cooked	125
Bass, steamed	120
Beans, baked in tomato sauce	75
French, green and runner	8
Haricot, other dried	75
Beef, hamburger, 1 medium	120
with roll	300
Oxtail stew	420
Sirloin, roast, lean	310
Steak, 8 oz. cooked	575
Steak and Kidney Pie	800
Stew with vegetables	600
Tongue, braised	380
Bitter Lemon, per glass	72
Beer, 1 large glass	180
Lager, 1 large glass	120
Blackberries, 1 bowl fresh	50
1 bowl stewed with sugar	150
Brains, raw or poached	115
Bran, per tblsp	5
Brandy, 1 measure	75
Bread, bread stick	15
Brioche, 1	225
Brown, 1 slice	68
Dinner roll	130
French, 2 small slices	125
Granary, 1 slice	65
Protein, 1 slice	50

92

Pumpernickel, 1 slice	75
Rye, 1 slice	65
White, 1 large slice.	100
Wholewheat	70
Breadcrumbs, 1 tsp.	10
Bread Pudding, 1 bowl.	250
Broccoli	25
Brussels sprouts.	40
Butter, 1 tblsp.	100
Cabbage, cooked	35
Red, pickled	50
Salad, cole slaw	50
Cakes, chocolate layer, 1 slice	450
Cheesecake, 1 square	460
Christmas cake, rich fruit	370
Gingerbread, 1 square	275
Sponge, 1 wedge.	125
with filling	450
Caramels, 1 square	100
Carrots, 1 raw	15
Cooked	45
Cauliflower, ...	25
with cheese sauce	280
Celery, 1 stick.	5
Celeriac, raw or boiled.	15
Champagne, dry, per glass	90
Sweet, per glass	120
Cheese, all 1 oz. portions	
Bel Paese	71
Brie.	90
Camembert	80
Cheddar.	108
Cottage	30
Cream	130
Danish Blue	110
Edam	95
Gouda	91
Gruyère	120
Parmesan.	30
Ricotta	75
Roquefort.	100
Swiss, 1 slice.	95
Cherries, raw, 1 bowl	100
in syrup.	250
Cherries glacé,1	15
Cherry Brandy, 1 glass	90
Chicken, roast, 1 portion	150
Dark meat only	170
White meat only	130
Chicken salad.	225
Chicory, raw.	10
Chocolate, milk, 1 bar	285
Plain, 1 bar, (small)	245
Unsweetened cooking, 1 square . .	150
Chocolate milk drink	250
Chutney, 1 tblsp.	25
Clams, with shells.	100
Clear soups, 1 bowl	40
Cocoa powder, 1 tblsp.	35
Coconut, shredded, 1 oz.	135
Cod, fillet, poached	80
fried fillet	325
Coffee, black	0
with cream.	30
Coffee with cream and sugar.	50
Cola drinks, 1 glass.	90
Low calorie drinks, 1 glass	1
Consommé, 1 bowl	24
Corn on the cob, 1 cob	75
Cornflakes, 1 bowl	100
Cranberry sauce, 1 tblsp.	35
Cream, 1 tblsp. thick	120
1 tblsp. thin	60
Crispbreads, 1 slice average.	25
Cucumbers, 1 whole raw	55
Currants, cooked with sugar	150
raw, 1 bowl	25
Dates, 1 whole.	17
Doughnut, jelly,1	200
Duck, roast, 1 portion	300

Eggs, 1 whole small	75
1 whole large	90
2 fried	300
2 scrambled	275
Figs, 1 raw	20
1 dried	65
Flounder, steamed	60
Fried	180
Flour, 1 tblsp.	38
Soya, 1 tblsp.	42
Frankfurter, 1 boiled	75
Fruit cocktail in syrup	250
Gin, 1 measure	70
Ginger, 1 piece crystallized.	120
Ginger ale, 1 glass	85
Dry ginger ale, 1 glass	24
Goose, roast, 1 portion.	325
Gooseberries, stewed with sugar, 1 bowl	100
Grapefruit, 1 half	50
in syrup, 1 bowl	120
Grapes, 1 small bunch	125
Greengages, 1 fresh	26
Haddock, fillet, 1 portion	125
smoked fillet	120
Fried fillet	300
Halibut, fillet, 1 portion.	150
Ham, baked, 1 portion.	370
Boiled no fat.	120
Steak, little fat	270
Herring, pickled,1.	25
Honey, 1 tsp.	20
Honeydew melon, 1 half	100
Ice cream, 1 scoop.	150
Jams & preserves, 1 tsp.	28
Kidneys, 2 average.	120
Lamb, roast, 1 portion	250
Chops, 2.	240
Stew, 1 bowl	490
Leeks, whole.	30
Lemon, 1 whole	30

Juice, 1 tblsp.	5
Lemon Meringue Pie.	230
Lemon Sole, portion	120
Lentil soup	315
Lentils, stewed	90
Lettuce, whole head	35
Liver, lamb or beef	120
Macaroni cooked.	120
Macaroons, 1.	45
Mackerel, 1 whole medium	150
Margarine, 1 tblsp.	100
Marmalade, 1 tsp.	25
Marshmallows, 2	50
Mayonnaise, 1 tblsp.	120
Melon, average half.	75
Milk, whole, 1 glass	160
Skimmed, 1 glass	100
Skimmed, powdered, 1 tblsp.	10
Evaporated, 1 tblsp.	30
Mushrooms, raw, 5	20
Fried.	75
Mushroom soup, 1 bowl	170
Mussels, 3 poached	8
Noodles, cooked, ...	120
Nuts, mixed, chopped, per tsp.	25
Oatmeal porridge, 1 bowl	75
Oil, salad, vegetable, 1 tblsp.	50
Olive, 1 tblsp.	120
Olives, 5 stoned	37
Onions, raw, 1 whole.	25
Orange, raw, 1 medium.	80
Juice, 1 glass.	110
Juice, per tblsp.	7
Oxtail soup, 1 bowl	200
Paté, 1 slice	110
Parsnips, boiled	50
Peach, raw, 1 whole.	50
in syrup, 2 halves	100
Peanut Butter, 1 tblsp.	175
Pear, raw, 1 medium	65

in syrup, 2 halves	100
Peas, raw or cooked.	60
Split or puréed	175
Peppers, green or red	30
Pineapple, 1 round slice	35
Plum, raw, 1 whole	20
Pork, roast, 1 portion	290
Chop, visible fat removed	190
Port, per glass.	135
Potatoes, baked, 1 whole	100
Boiled, portion	100
Fried, average portion	220
Salad, small scoop	170
Prawns and Shrimps.	90
Cocktail, with sauce.	200
Prunes, dried, 1 whole	15
Radish, 1 raw	2
Raisins, 2 tblsp.	60
Raspberries, 1 bowl	69
Rhubarb, 1 stick whole.	5
Cooked with sugar.	100
Rice, brown, cooked	115
White, cooked	130
Rum, 1 generous measure	110
Salmon, raw, 1 piece	175
Sardine, 1 in oil.	45
Sausages, assorted.	100
Sherry, 1 glass dry.	100
Soda-water, per glass	0
Spaghetti	225
with butter, cheese.	395
with tomato sauce, butter and	
cheese	450
Spinach, leaf	45
creamed.	125
Strawberries, 1 bowl.	35
with sugar and cream	210
Sugar, 1 tsp.	25
Sweetbreads, 2	125
Tangerine, 1 whole	45

Tea with Lemon.	0
with milk	25
Tomato, 1 whole	15
Purée, 1 tblsp.	25
Soup, 1 bowl	250
Tonic water, per glass	36
Trout, steamed 1 whole.	120
Turbot, steamed 1 slice	150
Tuna Fish, in oil.	250
Turkey, roast, 1 portion	200
Turnips.	50
Veal, roast.	485
Veal chop, lean	300
Shoulder, braised	480
Stew, with vegetables	650
Vegetable soup, clear	40
Thick with no potatoes	135
with potatoes and pasta	350
Venison, roast	200
Stew with vegetables.	480
Vodka, per glass	90
Walnuts, 15 shelled	450
1 nut	30
Watermelon, 1 slice.	100
Whiskies, 1 generous measure	100
Wine, dry red.	100
Dry, white	90

Low Calorie Menus

FAMILY		DIETER (1,200 Calories a Day)	
BREAKFAST	Fruit Juice Hot Porridge with Raisins Milk or Cream	**BREAKFAST**	Fruit Juice Special K Cereal with Raisins Skimmed Milk
LUNCH	Two-egg Omelet with Cheese Toast and Butter	**LUNCH**	Two-Egg Omelet with Cheese Thin Toast, 1 piece, no butter
DINNER	Beef Stew with Vegetables and Potatoes Green Salad, French Dressing Lemon and Orange Fluff (fruit juice, gelatine, sugar)	**DINNER**	Beef Stew with Vegetables (no potatoes, little gravy) Green Salad, Lemon Juice Lemon and Orange Fluff (with artificial sweetener)

BREAKFAST	¹/₂ Grapefruit Bacon and Tomato	**BREAKFAST**	¹/₂ Grapefruit 1 slice Bacon, 2 halves Tomato
LUNCH	Home-made Paté and Toast Gherkin Salad Cheese Board, Fresh Fruit	**LUNCH**	Home-made Paté, Celery Sticks Gherkin Salad Camembert or Edam, Apple
DINNER	Clear Chicken Soup, Noodles Poached Salmon, Mayonnaise Boiled Potatoes, Peas Peaches and Ice Cream	**DINNER**	Clear Soup and Sliced Mushrooms Poached Salmon with Lemon Peas, Cucumber Salad Peaches, no syrup

BREAKFAST	Fresh Berries and Cream Warm Rolls and Jam	**BREAKFAST**	Berries and Plain Yogurt Crispbread or Melba Toast
LUNCH	Thick Vegetable Soup with Macaroni French Bread, Butter	**LUNCH**	Thick Vegetable Soup (made without macaroni) Green or Mixed Salad
DINNER	Baked Pork Chops and Apple Glazed Onions, Baked Potato Raw Spinach Salad with Mushrooms Lemon Meringue Pie	**DINNER**	Baked Pork Chop (1) and Apple Glazed Onions, ¹/₂ Baked Potato Raw Spinach Salad with Mushrooms Edam or Gouda Cheese

FAMILY		DIETER	

BREAKFAST	Fried Eggs and Sausages Toast and Preserves	**BREAKFAST**	Poached Egg, 1 Sausage Crispbread, scraping Butter
LUNCH	Hamburger on Roll Fried Potatoes	**LUNCH**	Hamburger, no roll Raw Onion and Cucumber Salad
DINNER	Veal Cutlet coated in Egg and Breadcrumbs Herbed Carrots, Sauté Potatoes Sliced Tomato Salad Chocolate Pudding	**DINNER**	Veal Cutlet coated in dried onion and skim milk Herbed Carrots, Green Beans Sliced Tomato Salad Quartered Fresh Orange

BREAKFAST	1/2 Cantaloupe Melon Toast and Jams	**BREAKFAST**	1/4 Cantaloupe Melon Crispbread or Melba Toast (2)
LUNCH	Cheese Salad with Fresh Fruit Gooseberry Fool	**LUNCH**	Cottage Cheese with Grapefruit Sections
DINNER	Onion Soup with French Bread Baked Fish, Fresh Tomato Sauce Creamed Potatoes, Broccoli Green Salad, Italian Dressing Baked Gingered Rhubarb, with Custard	**DINNER**	Onion Soup (no bread) Baked Fish, Fresh Tomato Sauce Broccoli, Sliced Carrots Green Salad, Lemon Juice Rhubarb and Ginger with artificial sweetener, no custard

BREAKFAST	Hot Porridge or Muesli Stewed Prunes	**BREAKFAST**	Special K Cereal Stewed Prunes (4 only)
LUNCH	Grilled Cheese and Bacon Sandwich	**LUNCH**	Grilled Cheese and Bacon Sandwich on light or diet Bread
DINNER	Norwegian Fish Salad (herrings, sardines, pickles) Roast Chicken and Stuffing Roast Potatoes, Green Beans Red Pepper Salad Apple and Blackberry Pie	**DINNER**	Fish Salad, 3 herrings, 1 sardine, pickles Roast Chicken, white meat only, no stuffing, no skin Green Beans, Pepper Salad Fresh Apple

BREAKFAST	Pancakes with Syrup and Butter	**BREAKFAST**	Pancakes (2) with Fresh Fruit
LUNCH	Quick Rice Pilaf, with Diced Chicken and Green Pepper	**LUNCH**	Quick Rice Pilaf, small portion Green Salad
DINNER	Vegetable Platter with Mustard and Herb Sauces for dipping; Tomatoes, Cabbage, Broccoli, Mushrooms, Carrot Sticks, Onion Rings, Celery, Spinach, Crême Caramel	**DINNER**	Vegetable Platter as indicated, Lemon Quarters, little of the sauces Crême Caramel, no extra syrup

Low Carbohydrate Diet

LOW CARB COUNTING

Aside from calorie controlled diets, the most popular method of dieting is probably the carbohydrate controlled diet. It is a boon to anyone who likes a glass of wine with meals and can't be bothered to go through the tedious business of adding up calories. Here is the theory: cut way down on all foods that contain sugar or starch, and, provided the rest of your diet is reasonable (you don't go on an avocado binge or down six double whiskies) you will lose weight.

Although most of us eat about 16 ounces of carbohydrates a day we need only about 2 ounces. Provided you get this much, you prevent the build up of ketone bodies in the blood that you get on the all-protein diet. And although the weight loss will be slower, you have no problems from having to eliminate these excess wastes. On the carbohydrate controlled diet you generally lose weight rapidly at first (sometimes up to 8 pounds the first week!) then you reach a plateau for a while before you begin to lose again.

The reasons for reducing carbohydrates to lose weight are simple although carbohydrates are no more fattening than other foods. All foods contain calories and some, like fats, contain many more than starches and sugars. But carbohydrates often act as carriers – butter goes on the bread and the baked potato, so when you stop eating bread and potatoes, you automatically cut down on other high calorie foods as well. Since almost half of the calories in the average diet come from carbohydrate,

eliminating most of these foods from your diet quite naturally reduces your total calorie intake at the same time.

In theory, on this diet, you can have anything provided you count the grams of carbohydrate in everything that you eat. Keep the total for the day to a minimum (between 50 and 60 grams). In practice, being on a carbohydrate controlled diet usually means cutting out bread, milk, sugar, potatoes, ice cream, and sweet things. Eat moderate quantities of the leaf and bulb vegetables and fruits. Alcohol is not treated as a carbohydrate so you can allow yourself dry wines and distilled spirits in moderation (one of the reasons this diet is often called a diet for the drinking man). Of course, if you drink more you will not lose weight. They do have lots of calories.

Like the all-protein diet, this regime is not for someone who needs to reduce his cholesterol intake. And anyone following it must make sure to get enough vitamin C. Orange juice is fairly high in carbohydrate content; if you decide to omit it, then be sure you take a 100 milligram tablet of vitamin C each day. Liver is an excellent source of B complex vitamins, so it is good to eat it a couple of times a week if you can.

At first you will need to familiarize yourself with carbohydrate values of common foods. But this is easier to calculate than calories. Most foods fall into convenient categories, none, little, or a lot. Once you know them you will rarely have to look at a chart.

FOODS TO EAT IN UNLIMITED AMOUNTS

PROTEINS: beef, lamb, veal, liver, kidneys, chicken and turkey, pheasant, all kinds of fish, cheeses made from goats' milk, mozzarella, cottage cheese.

DRINKS: tea, coffee, calorie-free beverages

FOODS TO EAT IN MODERATE QUANTITIES

(Keep to less than 60 grams of carbohydrate – about 250 calories' worth a day)

FATS: Margarine, butter, cream, milk, oils.

EGGS

LEAFY VEGETABLES: Artichokes, asparagus, broccoli, cabbage, cauliflower, celery, chicory, kale, all kinds of lettuce and salad greens, spinach, watercress.

BULB VEGETABLES: Tomatoes, green and red peppers, cucumbers.

FRUITS: Lemons, oranges, grapefruit, tangerines, all kinds of berries.

DRY WINES: Red or white

DISTILLED SPIRITS: Whiskies, vodkas, gin

YOU NEED TO DRINK: 3 pints of water a day

THE GRAPEFRUIT DIET

Based on the low carbohydrate principle, this diet offers no magic despite all the mystique surrounding the idea that grapefruit is a slimming food. It is *not*. It is simply low in carbohydrates and provides necessary vitamins. But it is simple to follow either at home or in restaurants and is most effective after about a week.

BREAKFAST:
Half a grapefruit (unsweetened)
2 eggs cooked any style
2 slices of bacon
black coffee or tea (no milk, artificial sweetener if desired)

LUNCH AND DINNER:
Half a grapefruit
A modest portion of fish, meat or poultry
Salad with lemon juice dressing.
        or
Spinach and Broccoli
Coffee or tea

Carbohydrate Check

CARBOHYDRATE CHART

Most listings are for average servings – a usual serving of soup, two or three slices of meat, a spoonful or two of vegetables, a small bowl of berries or diced fruit, a middle-sized glass of about 7 or 8 ounces. Any other measurements are specified (a wedge of melon, one raw apple, etc.). Please remember that all numbers are approximate, since it is almost impossible to judge the exact size of a piece of fruit, or a spoonful of peas. So to be really strict with yourself, add up a slightly higher number of grams for each portion, and keep within your limit for the day – 30, if you are aiming for the quickest weight loss possible, 60, if you want to lose slowly but steadily. It's the same with all diets – if you pretend a large apple is a small one when you add up, then you're only fooling your mind, not your body.

There are no listings for negative carbohydrate foods – meat, fish (except for some seafoods which are listed), poultry, most fats and oils, hard liquors. When you are hungry, be sure you eat from the recommended listing — that includes snacks as well as meals!

This chart is comparatively short, but the foods have been chosen to give you a good representative selection of what may be part of your routine. There are whole booklets available listing almost every possible carbohydrate content.

Ale, 1 glass ($^1/_2$ pint tankard) 8.0
    Dark, 1 glass 10.2
Almonds, 15 whole 3.2

    1 Tblsp. chopped 1.9
Anchovies, 4 . . . . 0.1
Apple, 1 large fresh 24.0
    1 small fresh 12.6
    1 baked with sugar 48.0
    Cider, 1 glass 24.0
    Juice, 1 glass 35.0
    Pie, 1 2″ wedge 45.0
Apple sauce, unsweetened 8.7
Apricot, 3 medium fresh 14.2
    3–4 halves, syrup 25.1
    3–4 halves, dried 11.2
Artichoke, 1 whole boiled 12.7
    4 hearts 7.2
Asparagus, 5 medium spears 3.0
Avocado, $^1/_2$ medium 10.0
Banana, 1 medium 35.0
Barley, cooked 52.0
Barley & mushroom soup 00.0
Beans, baked 25.0
    Green, sliced 3.0
    Haricot, dried 28.0
    Various dried 31.0
Beer, 1 glass ($^1/_2$ pint) 11.0
Beets, cooked 14.0
    3 pickled, small 11.0
Benedictine, 1 liqueur glass 6.0
Biscuits, 1 sweet plain 0.0
    See also crackers, cookies
Blackberries 9.0
    See also Jams, Jellies
Blue cheese, 1 wedge 6.0
Bouillon, from cube 0.0
Brains 8.0
Bran Flakes 20.0
    Tblsp. unprocessed 5.0
Brazil nuts, 15 . . . . 6.0
Bread, French, Italian,
    Vienna, 1 small slice 10.0
    Granary, Cracked Wheat, Whole

Wheat, 1 slice 12.0
High protein, light or diet
type, 1 slice 8.0
Pumpernickel & rye, 1 slice 13.5
White, wrapped, 1 slice. 12.0
Bread crumbs, 1 Tblsp. 4.0
Bread stuffing, 1 Tblsp. 6.0
Brie cheese, 1 wedge. 0.0
Broccoli, 2–3 spears. 5.0
Brussels Sprouts 7.0
Buns, 1 plain sweet 20.0
Butter, 1 Tblsp. 0.1
Butterscotch, 1 square. 0.5
Cabbage, shredded raw 3.0
Shredded cooked 4.0
Chinese, shredded raw 1.5
Cake, plain sponge, 1 wedge 22.0
White layer, 3 layers 75.0
1 small iced square 32.0
See also individual types
Camembert, 1 triangle 0.5
Cantaloupe, $1/2$ melon 9.0
Caramel, 1 square. 8.0
Carrots, 1 raw 5.0
Cooked. 5.0
Juice, 1 glass 13.0
Cashew nuts, 15 . . . . 12.0
Cauliflower 3.0
Celery, 2 sticks. 3.0
Cereals, already sweetened 25.0–35.0
Corn Flakes 21.0
Muesli, commercial 32.0
Oatmeal, cooked 27.0
Rice Crispies. 25.0
Special K 12.0
Champagne, dry, 1 champagne
glass 2.0
Cocktail, 1 champagne glass 9.0
Chard, Swiss 3.2
Cheddar cheese, 1 ounce square 0.6

Cheesecake, 1 wedge or square 29.0
Cheese spreads, average 1
triangle 2.0
See also separate listings
Cherries, raw 6.9
Canned with syrup 30.0
Cherry brandy, 1 liqueur glass 6.0
Chutney, mango or fruit;
1 Tblsp. 10.0
Chocolate, 1 ounce square or bar. 8.0
Milk with nuts, 1 ounce 16.0
Creams, 1 piece. 9.0
Fudge, 1 square. 24.0
Layer cake, 3 layers. 63.0
Mint, 2 pieces thin squares 18.0
Brownie, 1 square 17.0
Clams, $1/2$ dozen 3.4
Clam chowder, New England 13.0
Cocoa, made with milk, 1 cup 25.0
Made $1/2$ milk, $1/2$ water, 1 cup 13.0
Cocoa powder, 1 Tblsp. 5.0
Coffee, one cup black 0.7
Coffeecake, 1 square average. 33.0
Colas, 1 glass 28.0
Colas, low calorie, 1 glass 0.0
Cottage Cheese, 1 small carton 2.5
Cole Slaw 0.0
Corn on the Cob, 1 ear 22.0
Chowder. 18.0
Creamed Kernels. 27.0
Crab, unshelled 0.8
Crackers, plain unsalted 7.0
Cheese and cocktail, 4 small. 1.2
Matzos and water. 7.0
Cranberries, raw 5.5
Jelly, 1 tsp. 3.0
Pie, 1 wedge 27.0
Juice, 1 small glass. 16.0
Cream (coffee), 1 Tblsp. 0.6
Whipping, 1 Tblsp. 0.4

Cream cakes, 1 slice 35.0–45.0	Lemon juice, 1 tsp. 1.2
Cream cheese, 1 Tblsp. 0.3	Meringue pie, 1 wedge 40.0
Crème de menthe, 1 liqueur glass 6.2	Lettuce, 1 head 14.0
Cucumber, 6 slices. 1.5	Lettuce & tomato salad 6.0
Custard, baked, 1 small cup 12.0	Liver, beef 6.0
Currants, dried, 1 Tblsp. 5.0	Calves 4.0
Red and black, fresh 8.0	Pork. 5.0
Dates, dried, 4. . . . . 28.0	Lentils, cooked 20.0
Egg, 1 medium 0.4	Soup 19.0
Endive, salad portion. 0.5	Macaroni, cooked. 16.0
Figs, fresh, 2 raw 20.0	Macaroon, 1 . . . . 14.0
dried, 2 . . . . 27.0	Marmalade, 1 tsp. 4.0
In syrup 24.0	Mayonaise, real, 1 tsp. 4.2
Fizzy sweet drinks, 1 glass 28.0	Milk, whole, 1 glass 12.0
Fruit cakes (raisin, currant,	Skim, 1 glass 13.0
etc.), 1 slice 23.0	Dry powder, skim, 1 tsp. 0.8
Fruit cocktail, fresh. 16.0	Mushrooms, 6 fresh 2.0
In syrup 24.0	Mussels, 1 dozen. 3.1
Fruit pies, average wedge 37.0	Noodles, egg, cooked 18.0
Fudge, assorted, 1 square 25.0	Olives, 5 large green 0.5
Fudge sauce, 1 Tblsp. 20.0	Onion, 1 large. 13.0
Ginger ale, 1 glass. 28.0	Chopped, 1 tsp. 0.5
Gingerbread, 1 square 27.0	Soup, with cheese 4.5
Ginger, candied, one small piece 27.0	Orange, 1 large. 28.0
Gooseberries, raw 7.0	1 small. 12.0
Grapefruit, $\frac{1}{2}$ medium 19.0	Juice, 1 small glass. 12.0
In syrup 24.0	Pancake, 1 6″ round 14.0
Grapes, 1 small bunch. 18.0	Parmesan cheese 1 tsp. grated 0.2
Gum drops 8.0	Parsnips. 10.0
Chewing gum, 1 stick 1.7	Pastries, French, 1 small. 25.0
Ham, baked with sugar. 0.5	Peach, 1 average raw 20.0
Hazelnuts, 15 . . . . 4.0	2 halves in syrup 25.0
Honeydew, $\frac{1}{4}$ melon 13.0	Nectar, 1 small glass 16.0
Hollandaise sauce. 0.0	Pear, 1 average raw 24.0
Ice cream, 1 scoop 6.0	2 halves in syrup 26.0
Ices and sherbets, 1 scoop. 13.0	Peanuts, 45 . . . . 4.0
Jams & Jellies, 1 tsp. 4.0–5.0	Peanut brittle, 1 piece 21.0
Kale, cooked. 4.0	Peanut butter, 1 Tblsp. 4.0
Kidneys, lamb 1.0	Peas, green raw. 11.0
Leeks, 2 large 6.0	Split, cooked 22.0

Soup 17.0	Stewed as vegetable. 4.0
Pecans, 15. . . . . 2.0	Tongue, 2 slices. 0.3
Pecan Pie, 1 wedge. 61.0	Tonic water, 1 glass 9.0
Peppers, green & red, 1 medium 3.0	Turnips 4.5
Pickle, dill, 1 medium. 2.0	Vermouth, dry, 1 small glass 0.1
Pickle relish, 1 tsp. 1.2	Sweet, 1 small glass. 12.0
Pies, 2 crust average 48.0	Vinegar, 1 tsp. 0.2
1 crust average 39.0	Vinegar and oil dressing, 1 tsp 3.0
See also individual listing	Walnuts, 15 halves 3.1
Pie crust only, 1 triangle 9.0	Watercress, few sprigs. 0.2
Pineapple, fresh, 1 slice 12.0	Soup, cream of 12.0
2 slices in syrup 30.0	Wine, dry table, 1 wineglass 0.5
Pistachios, 15 . . . . 1.2	Sweet table, 1 wineglass. 5.0
Plum, 1 medium 7.0	
4 halves in syrup 19.0	
Plum pudding, 1 slice 48.0	
Potato, 1 medium cooked. 23.0	
Potato salad 14.0	
Port, 1 small glass 6.0	
Prunes, 6 dried. 35.0	
Radish, 3 small 1.5	
Raisins, dried, 1 Tblsp. 5.0	
Rice, cooked, white or brown 22.0	
Rhubarb, cooked without sugar 3.0	
Cooked with sugar 50.0	
Rolls, dinner. 17.0	
Hamburger size. 21.0	
Russian dressing 1.5	
Russian salad. 15.0	
Scotch broth 9.0	
Sherry, 1 sherry glass 5.0	
Shrimp, 6 large 2.4	
6 large breaded 8.5	
Spinach, leaf, cooked 5.9	
Creamed. 9.0	
Sugar, brown, 1 tsp. 4.5	
White, 1 tsp. 4.0	
Swiss cheese, 1 thin slice 0.5	
Tomato, 1 medium. 6.0	
Tomato purée, 1 tsp 0.1	

Low Carbohydrate Menu

Remember that all diets which eliminate or cut down drastically on any one group of foods are not for long-term good health.

The very low carbohydrate count of 30 grams a day which is sometimes recommended is only for short periods, and never for more than a few weeks unless you have a doctor's approval. Even counting 60 grams, it is probably better to stay on it for no more than a few weeks at any one time.

FAMILY

BREAKFAST	Fruit Juice Eggs and Bacon
LUNCH	Fisherman's Salad French Bread
DINNER	Meat Loaf (all meat, no cereal) Green Beans, Mushrooms Baked Potatoes Fresh Fruit Salad, Cream

BREAKFAST	Cornflakes and Stewed Fruit Toast and Jam
LUNCH	Salade Niçoise, (made with tuna fish, olives, anchovies)
DINNER	Chicken in Wine and Mushroom Sauce, Sauté Potatoes Creamed Spinach, Coleslaw Cheese Board, Celery Sticks

BREAKFAST	Ham Omelet Rolls and Butter
LUNCH	Cottage Cheese and Fruit Salad
DINNER	Braised Beef with Gravy Egg Noodles Broccoli, Carrots Orange Meringue Pudding

DIETER

BREAKFAST	$\frac{1}{2}$ Grapefruit Eggs and Bacon
LUNCH	Fisherman's Salad Small Green Salad
DINNER	Meat Loaf Green Beans, small portion Mushrooms, very small portion

BREAKFAST	Slice of Meat Loaf, with Poached Egg
LUNCH	Salad Niçoise, mostly fish
DINNER	Chicken without extra sauce small Coleslaw Salad Square of Hard Cheese

BREAKFAST	Ham Omelet
LUNCH	Cold Chicken and small Salad
DINNER	Braised Beef, no gravy, no noodles small portion Broccoli Macaroon (1 small)

FAMILY		DIETER	

BREAKFAST	Bacon, Sausage, Tomato Toast and Marmalade	**BREAKFAST**	Bacon and Sausage (pure meat only)
LUNCH	Welsh Rarebit on Cauliflower	**LUNCH**	Welsh Rarebit on Poached Eggs
DINNER	Roast Leg of Lamb with Garlic and Parsley Sauce Roast Potatoes, Puréed Peas Leaf Spinach, Mixed Salad Cooked Fresh Pears	**DINNER**	Roast Leg of Lamb with a little Garlic Sauce small portion Spinach small Mixed Salad Square of hard cheese

BREAKFAST	½ Grapefruit Muesli and Grated Apple	**BREAKFAST**	Cold Ham and mustard
LUNCH	Cold Lamb and Chutney	**LUNCH**	Cold Lamb, no chutney
DINNER	Clear Soup with Rice Fish Fillets with Spicy Tomato Sauce Fried Potatoes, Corn on the Cob Mint Chocolate Fluff made with artificial sweetener and gelatine	**DINNER**	Clear Soup, no Rice Fish Fillets, Lemon Slices Herb Tea

BREAKFAST	Hot Porridge and Cream Toast and Preserves	**BREAKFAST**	Fish Fillets with Salad Dressing
LUNCH	Chicken Salad Mixed Bean Garnish	**LUNCH**	Chicken Salad
DINNER	Chicken Soup with Dumplings Steak and Kidney Pie Brussels Sprouts, Carrots Cheese Board, Fresh Fruit	**DINNER**	Chicken Soup, no dumplings Steak and Kidney, no pastry small portion Carrots Square of hard cheese

BREAKFAST	Kippered Herring Fillets Tomato Halves, Toast	**BREAKFAST**	Kippered Herring Fillets Poached Egg
LUNCH	Home-made Paté French Bread	**LUNCH**	Paté with its Chopped Jelly
DINNER	Loin of Pork with Prunes Boiled Potatoes Braised Red Cabbage Green Pepper Salad Lemon Pudding	**DINNER**	Loin of Pork, cut very lean small portion Pepper Salad Herb Tea

105

All-Protein Diet

AN EASY DIET TO FOLLOW

The formula is simple: eat no carbohydrates, no fats, only high protein foods and drink lots of water. How much you eat is up to you but you will lose weight more rapidly if you eat only enough to satisfy your hunger and don't simply indulge in eating for the sake of it.

Often called the 'Stillman Diet' after the doctor who popularized it, it depends for its effectiveness on a rather complex and unnatural effect that eating solely protein foods has on the body.

Protein has the ability to increase the rate of metabolism. It also takes longer and requires more calories to digest than either starches or fats. On this diet, in the process of digestion alone, you will use up an additional 275 calories a day over any other diet that offers the same number of calories but which includes foods containing fats and carbohydrates too. Protein foods like meat, fish, and poultry are also stimulants that give you a feeling of lift, helping you to avoid the tired feeling that can sometimes go along with strict dieting.

Usually the body relies for its energy on carbohydrates, that is, starches and sugars. When you eat only high protein foods, it has to use up stored fat both for energy and in order to help digest and metabolize the food eaten. Sixty per cent of this fat, which is drawn from the body's reserves, will be completely oxidized (turned into carbon dioxide and water) and disappear in the process. The rest, however, remains in the body to be disposed of in the form of unused fatty acids such as oxybutyric and acetoacetic acid, sometimes called ketone bodies. Ketones are like clinkers left in a furnace, and they need to be washed out of the system. The body withdraws water from the cells to do the job.

This often means frequent urination on the all protein diet, and considerable water loss from the tissues, a boon to anyone who tends to suffer from water retention.

But unfortunately, it is not all so rosy as it sounds. These clinkers are after all, the product of incomplete oxidation and cause irritation to the kidneys and the liver, the two organs which they pass through while in the urine. In a young healthy body this is usually not too much trouble, but as the body grows older, the elimination processes are not so efficient. So if you stayed on all proteins for a long time, it could lead to a concentration of these acid wastes in the system, and increased acidity of the blood and urine. This may be particularly bad for people with a tendency towards rheumatism, arthritis, or gout. The diet is also not generally recommended by doctors for anyone who should avoid high-cholesterol foods.

At any age, a long period on this kind of diet puts a definite strain on the body, particulary the kidneys and liver, and may contribute to the development of other health problems, too. So be sensible; — it does work quickly, and you can alternate 2 or 3 weeks on all-proteins with a similar period on a better-balanced, low-calorie diet.

It is essential that there are no slips. Even *one*

mouthful of ice cream, or a chocolate bar, or an apple, will set you back a couple of days. If you disregard the formula and eat carbohydrates, sugar or alcohol regularly you will simply stop the efficient fat-burning process and stop losing weight.

WHAT TO EAT

LEAN MEATS: boiled, baked or grilled but not cooked in butter or other fat. Trim all excess fat from meat before cooking.

LEAN FISH AND SHELL FISH: again boiled, grilled or baked without excess fat. No tartar sauce or mayonaise.

POULTRY: Grilled, boiled or baked without extra fat. Remove skin before eating.

COTTAGE CHEESE AND FARMERS CHEESE: very low in fat, or fat-free, varieties only.

EGGS: preferably hard-boiled, but can be cooked in other ways provided you use no fat in cooking.

A MULTIPLE VITAMIN-MINERAL CAPSULE: this supplies the nutrients you may be missing from eliminating grains, fruits and vegetables.

DRINKS: as much tea and coffee as you like but unsweetened and without milk or cream. (You may use artificial sweeteners if you wish). All non-caloric carbonated drinks.

YOU MUST DRINK AT LEAST 6–8 GLASSES OF WATER A DAY. YOU MUST EAT NOTHING ELSE.

SLIGHTLY LESS SEVERE

A variation of the All Protein Diet theme is the Protein-Fat-Salad Diet. It can be used after the first two or three weeks particularly successfully. Its working principles are the same. It is still very low in carbohydrates and also gives a steady weight loss although this will be slower than on the pure protein regime. It is particularly good for some people who find they are irritable if they take no fat in their diet. In addition to the foods already listed you may eat:

HARD CHEESE: Cheddar, parmesan, etc.
FATS: Butter, margarine, oils and cream (but no milk)
SALAD: One small green portion with each meal
FRUIT: The juice of one lemon each day.

You can grill or bake your foods or cook them in a pan on the stove in a little fat. You must still drink the three pints of water and take a multiple vitamin-mineral supplement each day.

Avoid citrus fruit, except for the lemon juice.

All-Protein Menus

FAMILY		DIETER	

FAMILY

BREAKFAST Tomato or Fruit Juice
Cornflakes and Stewed Prunes

LUNCH Cheeseburgers on a Roll
Pickles and Salad

DINNER Curried Lamb New Delhi
Brown Rice Pilaf
Chopped Cucumber in Yoghurt
Ice Cream and Ginger Sauce

DIETER

BREAKFAST Cold Meat, mustard (remove all fat)
Vitamin supplement

LUNCH Hamburger (no cheese, hamburger made without cereal or flour)

DINNER Curried Lamb without sauce
Herb Tea

BREAKFAST Sliced Oranges
Boiled Eggs
Wholewheat Toast and Butter

LUNCH Cold Meat Platter and Salad

DINNER Mediterranean Fish Casserole
Garlic Bread
Green Bean Salad
Cheese Board and Fresh Fruit

BREAKFAST Boiled Eggs
Vitamin supplement

LUNCH Cold Meat Platter

DINNER Fish Casserole
Herb Tea

BREAKFAST $1/2$ Grapefruit
Smoked Haddock

LUNCH Cheddar Cheese Soup
Crusty Rolls

DINNER Barbecued Chicken
and Mushroom Gravy
Creamed Spinach, Carrots
Green Salad, French Dressing
Lemon Pudding

BREAKFAST Smoked Haddock
Vitamin supplement

LUNCH Cold Fish with Lemon Dressing

DINNER Barbecuea Chicken
Herb Tea

FAMILY		DIETER	

	FAMILY		DIETER
BREAKFAST	Oatmeal and Grated Apple	**BREAKFAST**	Cold Chicken Pieces Vitamin Supplement
LUNCH	Cottage Cheese and Tomato	**LUNCH**	Cottage Cheese
DINNER	Crisp-Fried Pork Chops Fried Rice Steamed Broccoli and Soy Sauce Pea Pods and Mushrooms Bananas and Cream	**DINNER**	Baked Pork Chops, trimmed of all fat Herb Tea

	FAMILY		DIETER
BREAKFAST	Orange Juice Scrambled Eggs and Bacon	**BREAKFAST**	Scrambled Eggs and Bacon Vitamin supplement
LUNCH	Fish Chowder French Bread	**LUNCH**	Fish Chowder
DINNER	Spinach and Cheese Quiche Baked Potatoes Sliced Tomatoes and Cucumber Hot Dried Apricot Salad	**DINNER**	Any lean meat (steak, liver) Herb Tea

	FAMILY		DIETER
BREAKFAST	Fruit Juice Sausage and Tomato	**BREAKFAST**	Sausage and Eggs (pure-meat sausage only) Vitamin supplement
LUNCH	Tuna Fish Salad	**LUNCH**	Tuna Fish and Cottage Cheese
DINNER	Consommé with Noodles Roast Beef in Pastry Roast Potatoes Peas and Onions Pineapple Upside Down Cake	**DINNER**	Consommé without noodles Roast Beef, no Pastry Herb Tea

	FAMILY		DIETER
BREAKFAST	Cheese and Chive Omelet Toast and Preserves	**BREAKFAST**	Ham Omelet Vitamin supplement
LUNCH	Cold Beef and Salad	**LUNCH**	Cold Beef and Mustard
DINNER	Chicken Stew with Vegetables Boiled Potatoes Green Salad and French Dressing Oranges in Caramel Sauce	**DINNER**	Chicken Stew Herb Tea

High Protein Menus

FAMILY		DIETER	
BREAKFAST	Tomato or Fruit Juice Cornflakes and Stewed Prunes	**BREAKFAST**	High Protein Cereal, Skim Milk
LUNCH	Cheeseburgers on a Roll Pickles and Salad	**LUNCH**	Cheeseburger, no roll 1 Pickle
DINNER	Curried Lamb New Delhi Brown Rice Pilaf Chopped Cucumber in Yoghurt Ice Cream and Ginger Sauce	**DINNER**	Curried Lamb, no gravy Cucumber, small portion Apple or Pear

BREAKFAST	Sliced Oranges Boiled Eggs Wholewheat Toast and Butter	**BREAKFAST**	Sliced Oranges Boiled Eggs Wholewheat Toast, 1 slice
LUNCH	Cold Meat Platter and Salad	**LUNCH**	Cold Meat Platter, no salad
DINNER	Mediterranean Fish Casserole Garlic Bread Green Bean Salad Cheese Board and Fresh Fruit	**DINNER**	Mediterranean Fish Casserole Green Bean Salad Lemon Juice Dressing Skim Milk Cheese

BREAKFAST	$^1/_2$ Grapefruit Smoked Haddock	**BREAKFAST**	$^1/_2$ Grapefruit Smoked Haddock
LUNCH	Cheddar Cheese Soup Crusty Rolls	**LUNCH**	Square of Cheddar Cheese High Protein Bread, 2 slices
DINNER	Barbecued Chicken and Mushroom Gravy Creamed Spinach, Carrots Green Salad, French Dressing Lemon Pudding	**DINNER**	Barbecued Chicken, no gravy Leaf Spinach Salad with Bacon Lemon Juice Dressing Herb Tea

FAMILY		DIETER	

BREAKFAST	Oatmeal and Grated Apple	**BREAKFAST**	Cold Chicken Pieces
LUNCH	Cottage Cheese and Tomato	**LUNCH**	Cottage Cheese and Tomato
DINNER	Crisp-Fried Pork Chops Fried Rice Steamed Broccoli and Soy Sauce Pea Pods and Mushrooms Bananas and Cream	**DINNER**	Crisp-Fried Pork Chops, (trimmed all fat) no rice Small portion Broccoli Camembert Cheese

BREAKFAST	Orange Juice Scrambled Eggs and Bacon	**BREAKFAST**	Orange Juice Scrambled Eggs and Bacon
LUNCH	Fish Chowder French Bread	**LUNCH**	Fish Chowder Wholewheat Toast, 1 slice
DINNER	Spinach and Cheese Quiche Baked Potatoes Sliced Tomatoes and Cucumber Hot Dried Apricot Salad	**DINNER**	Spinach and Cheese Quiche without pastry Small portion Salad Herb Tea

BREAKFAST	Fruit Juice Sausage and Tomato	**BREAKFAST**	Grapefruit Juice Sausage and Eggs
LUNCH	Tuna Fish Salad	**LUNCH**	Tuna Fish Salad
DINNER	Consommé with Noodles Roast Beef in Pastry Roast Potatoes Peas and Onions Pineapple Upside Down Cake	**DINNER**	Consommé without noodles Roast Beef, no Pastry Peas and Onions, small portion Pineapple, 1 slice

BREAKFAST	Cheese and Chive Omelet Toast and Preserves	**BREAKFAST**	Cheese and Chive Omelet High Protein Bread, 1 slice
LUNCH	Cold Beef and Salad	**LUNCH**	Cold Beef and Mustard
DINNER	Chicken Stew with Vegetables Boiled Potatoes Green Salad and French Dressing Oranges in Caramel Sauce	**DINNER**	Chicken Stew Green Salad, Lemon Juice and Herb Dressing Oranges, no Sauce

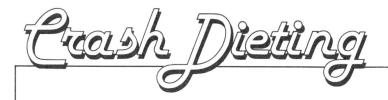

Crash Dieting

QUICK AND EASY

A crash diet to lose weight quickly can be a boon or a bane, depending on what it is, and how it is used. Going onto crash diets constantly and gorging yourself in between is no way to stay healthy. See-sawing up and down can even do a considerable amount of damage to your whole system. The skin stretches and contracts too quickly, so that it gets out of shape, and loses elasticity; an uneven supply of vitamins and minerals may lead to deficiencies, lack-lustre hair, splitting nails, and stomach and digestive problems.

The quickly-added weight that piles back on during the no-diet period may encourage serum cholestrol to build up in the lung and heart system. And the level may not drop back to normal when the pounds come off again.

Some of the crash diets suggested by magazines and articles are enough to curl the hair of any nutritionist, although they may be temporarily effective. A wine diet of hard-boiled eggs and wine for breakfast, lunch, and dinner isn't really well-balanced, although it may help you to become an expert on vintage bottling!

Basically a crash diet should use a minimal amount of food, and only those foods which can give you enough nourishment to keep going for a period, without putting too much strain on your body.

Quick and easy, it's the preliminary kick-off to a long diet plan. Because the results are usually immediate and quite dramatic, it acts like a mental tonic, and convinces you that dieting really works. You are off to a good start, and already accustomed to eating less.

Then, a carefully controlled crash diet can act something like a fast, benefiting your overall vitality, and making your eyes and skin look bright and clear.

It is this second effect which keeps business booming at exclusive health resorts, where clients come from all over the world to be re-vitalized and pampered. That's something we all enjoy, and though going to a health farm is out of reach for most of us with daily responsibilities, then we can make our own treatments at home.

The diets we suggest here are not just fads dreamed up for publicity. They have all been used for many years, and have individual benefits which might help your particular problem, as well as taking off a few pounds.

If you plan to go on a crash diet, then at least take it seriously. Plan ahead so you won't have to go out to a party on the second night, or you'll be sorely tempted to undo all the good work.

And plan enough time for yourself, even if it's only this once.

Do check with your doctor before you begin, and do not exceed the number of days we suggest. These are short term quick working tonics for your body, not plans for lasting good health.

Later, go back to eating gradually, with light, small snacks on the first day. A huge dinner of lobster in cream sauce will be too rich, and it will probably make you sick.

HOW TO USE CRASH DIETING SUCCESSFULLY

CHOOSE YOUR DIET WELL so it fits in with your personal tastes, your lifestyle and offers a particular bonus like water loss from the tissues if you tend to retain water, or restoring good elimination if you tend to be constipated.

PLAN YOUR TIME so that you can handle the demands and fit them into your family life, at work, or at home. If you don't you will probably break your regime as suddenly as you began it.

DON'T WORRY IF YOU'RE TIRED, a bit headachey or feel a little unwell sometime in the first two or three days. This is the result of a drastic change in food intake that sparks off rapid elimination of stored wastes from the body. Do nothing but rest more if you can, and it will pass naturally as your body becomes used to the new regime.

GET SOME DAILY EXERCISE. It will help in the slimming and toning-up process. Try to walk for 30 minutes twice a day.

TRY TO REST a bit more than usual. Go to bed early and, if possible, lie down for 10 to 20 minutes in the afternoon.

GET YOUR DOCTOR'S APPROVAL before you begin.

Crash Diet Menus

ORANGE AND ONION DIET

Good for people who would like to fast, but can't because they are working. It gives the system a really massive cleanout, and it's an excellent start to a long term reducing plan. If you can stay on it for five to seven days, you could lose up to 10 or 12 pounds.

BREAKFAST

One to three oranges

LUNCH

Onions baked in their skins, or steamed in a minimum of water – drink the water, too. You may have two or three large ones each meal.

AFTERNOON BREAK

Same as breakfast.

DINNER

Same as lunch.

Use herbs in cooking onions if you wish, and drink water, herb teas without milk or sweeteners, or mineral water between meals. Try to last at least one hour before and after meals without additional liquid. During this diet never drink at meal times, except for the juice from the onions, or the natural orange juice.

THE ALL FRUIT DIET

It is good for eliminating excess catarrh, useful for high blood pressure sufferers, people with muscle and joint aches, and as a general clean out, it is also good for getting rid of that jaded feeling that comes after a period of over-indulgence in food and alcohol. It can be easily followed if you have to eat in a restaurant; stay on it no more than five days, to lose up to eight pounds.

BREAKFAST

An orange or half a grapefruit

LUNCH

Fresh fruit salad (no added sugar) or assorted fresh fruit (melon, cherries, apples, oranges, mangos, pawpaw, berries, pineapple).

DINNER

As lunch. You can add cinnamon to the salad to add to the taste.

DRINKS

Herb teas (without milk, but sweetened with honey if desired), water, mineral waters, nothing else.

VARIATION: THE GRAPE CURE

Eat four pounds of fresh grapes each day. They can be white or red and eaten at any time you wish throughout the day. Be sure to wash them thoroughly and eat the whole grape, skin, pips, and all. You may have the drinks listed above, nothing else.

THE LASSI LIQUID DIET

Good for a long weekend rest from solid food. No more than three days, and you'll lose up to five pounds.

FORMULA

To two pints of skimmed milk, add 8 ounces of natural yogurt, two eggs, the juice of three oranges, 1 tablespoon of olive, corn or sunflower seed oil, 2 tablespoons of honey, and half a teaspoon of vanilla extract. Mix well in a blender. You may season the lassi with a little ground cinnamon, mace, corriander or mixed spice if desired.

JUICE-SALAD-YOGURT DIET

A 'spring-cleaning' diet, this is excellent at the change of the season to give you a feeling of renewed vigor, brighten dull looking skin, and re-educate your eating habits if you have been on a diet too rich in protein or refined carbohydrates. You can stay on this for up to ten days to lose about 12 pounds.

BREAKFAST
7 ounces of unsweetened freshly made fruit juice. It can be orange or grapefruit or, if you have a centrifuge juice extractor, any of the following either in combination or on their own: apple, grape, pineapple, cherry, berry, melon, peach. 5 ounces of natural unsweetened yogurt.

LUNCH
A raw vegetable plate made from one leaf vegetable (lettuce, endive, cabbage, cress, watercress, corn salad, chicory), one bulb vegetable (tomato, cucumber, bell peppers, celery, fennel) and one root vegetable (celeriac, carrot, salsify, radishes, beets, kohlrabi). You may add a little oil and lemon dressing made with fresh or dried herbs and then sprinkle with 2 tablespoons of chopped mixed raw nuts such as Brazils, hazelnuts, cashews, almonds, or sunflower seeds. (They can be easily chopped in a coffee grinder or blender and kept in the refrigerator.)

Store in the refrigerator and drink as you wish throughout the day. You may also have water, mineral water and herb tea sweetened with a little honey and with milk if desired.

DINNER
Same as breakfast, or you can substitute two pieces of fresh fruit. (Lunch and dinner are interchangeable but it is better to have the larger meal at noon, if possible).

DRINKS
Herb teas; (try camomile for relaxing, mint for a boost, solidago (also called golden rod) or nettle if you usually retain water, mineral water, water. Nothing else.

NOTE
The elimination process is helped by brushing your skin before a bath every day with a loofah or hemp glove and exercising moderately. No strenuous exercise like tennis or squash unless you are already used to it.

THE MILK DIET

This diet encourages the elimination of excess fluids from the body by stimulating the kidneys. It is useful for people with minor skin troubles, stomach complaints, and those who retain fluids. Not for more than three or four days, and you should lose five pounds.

FORMULA
Each day drink four glasses of milk, either on its own or mixed with sparkling mineral water such as Vichy (one litre a day). Nothing else.

VARIATION
Milk is made more digestible by adding the juice of half a lemon to a pint of boiled milk which curdles. A tablespoon of honey can also be added for sweetening if desired. Nothing else but pure water.

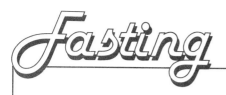
Fasting

NO FOOD AT ALL

Fasting is a remarkable tool which has been used for almost every human purpose, from religious ritual to losing weight, clearing out debris from the body, and helping to cure many ailments, both mental and physical. Fasting is also highly controversial, and often misunderstood, something that one should never do for more than a day or a few days at the most except under medical supervision. And remember fasting means going without food, never *never* without liquids. Any restriction of liquids when fasting is DANGEROUS.

The practice of temporarily refusing food is ancient. Socrates fasted to improve his mental clarity; Persian and Greek physicians used it to cure illnesses from syphillis to general debility, while mystics of all the world's religions have talked about fasting as a way of expanding spiritual awareness, or cutting us off the overdependence on the material aspects of life.

There are more practical uses, too; some doctors in Europe and America now use fasting successfuly to treat such things as resistant obesity, bronchitis, anaemia, migraines, high blood pressure, and arthritis. Russian doctors have reported excellent results, treating schizophrenia and other forms of severe mental illness even where other forms of treatment have failed. Yet many people still dismiss the idea of no food completely, claiming that it is dangerous not to eat, even for short periods. It seems a pity, because most of us would surely find it helpful to give our digestive systems a rest. There are exceptions, of course, set out clearly on the next page.

The technique of fasting is not complicated. You simply stop eating and go without food until your doctor tells you it is time to eat again. A short fast of two or three days for a healthy person usually has no complications. During a true fast, you drink nothing but water, with or without a vitamin and mineral supplement. Modified fasts, where you drink fruit or vegetable juices, are also used, particularly for people who are frightened of going without food completely. In recent years the protein sparing diet has become popular, where a five-ounce supplement of liquid amino acids supplies from 300 to 360 calories a day, and it has been used for dieting, too. But this requires supervision – never to be used without medical advice.

A properly supervised fast should never be dangerous. If you are very thin restrict your days without food to only one or two a month. If you are in good health, normal weight, or overweight you can safely fast for from several days to even several weeks, but only under a doctor's supervision.

According to experts on fasting, the positive effects are improved health and a feeling of vitality, and these are the result of a drastic elimination of stored wastes or toxins from the system. Fasting also gives the body a rest from having to process large quantities of food – and tends to lower blood cholestrol levels. During a fast your body lives on its own energy supply, breaking down stored fat in the tissues, metabolizing it and eliminating waste products, at the same time. Most chemical pollutants in the air or on our foods such as DDT are also stored in the fat cells of the body; as the fat breaks down pollutants are also eliminated.

This process results in a kind of rejuvenation, and a generally youthful sensation. Many women find after a fast that the fine lines of their face have softened, muscles appear firmer and they look younger. For this reason they fast 2 or 3 days a month or even a week. Fasting also appears to encourage the more rapid repair of damage in the body. A cut will heal more quickly than usual during a fast.

From the time that the first meal is skipped, the profound process of elimination begins. Occasionally fasters experience a slight feeling of sickness or a headache on the first or second day, but that passes quickly. After two or three days the feeling of hunger disappears and doesn't return again until the body's fat reserves are used up.

If you are a young mother with babies or toddlers, one day is probably all you should manage. Concentrate on keeping to a reasonable diet instead. One word of warning here, especially to mothers of teenage girls. Sometimes the realization that it is possible to go without food triggers off the first symptoms of anorexia nervosa. If you've ever had a problem with yourself or your daughter about excessive dieting, then it would be better to avoid fasting altogether. Even crash diets might be too severe. Go to see your doctor, and listen to his advice – anorexia is a growing problem.

But if you are generally in good health, if you keep to the rules for sensible fasting, and if you have your doctor's approval, then giving your whole body a rest a few times a year should benefit every part of your system.

THE BASIC WATER FAST

Never use it for longer than two or three days without close medical supervision. This is true fasting.

Spend as much time as possible doing quiet, pleasant things such as going for long walks, reading or listening to music. It often brings a sense of inner calm and contentment.

FORMULA:
Drink as much as you want (but at least six glasses a day) of pure, preferably spring water. (Vital, Vichy, Evian, etc).

ELEVEN RULES TO FOLLOW

1. GET YOUR DOCTOR'S APPROVAL. Don't fast if you are pregnant, a nursing mother, or have any of the following ailments: juvenile diabetes, kidney diseases, liver diseases, gout, active pulmonary illnesses, bleeding ulcers, cancer, heart disease (especially a predisposition to thrombosis), recent myocardial infarction or cerebral diseases. Don't fast if you are on drug therapy of any kind.

2. GET ENOUGH REST. Choose a time when you have no heavy work and can rest and sleep when you feel like it. Go to bed early when you can and try to rest for 10 to 15 minutes in the middle of the day if possible.

3. EAT SPARSELY for a couple of days before you begin, preferably a diet of raw fruits and vegetables which will begin the clean-out process and make the fast easier.

4. DON'T DRINK COFFEE, TEA OR ALCOHOL during a fast. You could undo all the good you have done.

5. TAKE PLENTY OF BATHS. They are refreshing, and help clear away the toxins released through the pores of the skin.

6. TAKE LIGHT EXERCISE. Walking is good, but no strenuous physical exercise unless you are used to it.

7. CARRY A TOOTHBRUSH with you. Your breath may smell differently at the beginning of the fast while your body is throwing off waste products at an enormous rate.

8. KEEP WARM. While fasting you can feel chillier than usual. Carry an extra sweater.

9. SPEND SOME TIME ON YOURSELF. Fasters claim they have an increased sense of inner calm they don't ordinarily experience. Enjoy it. Any fast is an ideal time to be self-indulgent. Let the children cook their own dinners, make their own sandwiches. Pour bath oil and scent into the bath, cream yourself all over, do light stretching exercises. Cream your face night and morning and give yourself a rest from make-up.

10. AVOID ALARMISTS like the plague. There is nothing worse than well-meaning relatives who telephone every few hours with questions. Remember, nothing dreadful is going to happen to you, regardless of their worries. Even the most sceptical physicians admit that a short fast of two or three days is harmless, even helpful, as most of us tend to eat far too much too often.

11. BREAKING YOUR FAST. Go back to eating slowly, with small, light meals of soup, vegetables and fruit, to give your body time to re-adjust.

THE JUICE FAST

The juice fast is useful for someone who wants to fast but has to be physically active, working or caring for a family. Its action on the body is not quite as drastic in terms of elimination as true fasting. This regime is also helpful when you are stuck in bed with flu, a cold, or other minor illnessess.

Raw juices are rich in vitamins, minerals, trace elements and enzymes all of which are easily assimilated when taken in liquid form. Ideally the juices should be made and drunk immediately.

MORNING:
8 ounces of fresh fruit juice mixed with an equal amount of water and sipped slowly (preferably from a spoon like soup).

LUNCHTIME:
8 ounces of vegetable juice (carrot, tomato or mixed vegetables) diluted with an equal amount of water. Sip slowly.

AFTERNOON:
Same as breakfast.

EVENING:
Same as lunchtime.

You may also drink unsweetened herb teas and pure water at any time during the day. Nothing else.

LEMON AND MOLASSES FAST

This fast is good for cleaning out the digestive system and for those who have a tendency towards constipation. After two or three days the body assimilates nutrients from food more easily when the fast is broken.

FORMULA:
Mix 2 tablespoons of fresh lemon juice with 2 tablespoons of blackstrap molasses. Add six cups of hot, pure water. Drink this mixture six times a day.

The molasses is a rich source of minerals (including iron) and has a natural laxative effect on the system. The lemon juice is to help neutralize the acids thrown into the bloodstream from the fast. Take nothing else except pure water.

Underweight

PUTTING IT ON

Although it seems incredible to those who always seen to be fighting the battle of the bulges, gaining weight can be a great problem. Being too thin means worrying about not eating, trying to eat too much, feeling sick, and worrying more, in an awful vicious circle!

The problem can be really difficult, particularly if 'skinny' is a child with parents who anxiously equate chubbiness with health. Surely there must be something wrong with a bean pole! But if the doctor has said all is well, then it's time to be thankful. For an adult, though there is an important question to ask before concentrating on trying to gain: am I *really* too thin? Or is my worry perhaps an attention-getting device? This can be especially true of women who desperately want to curve in all the feminine places. Men, too, peek at body-building ads, and look in the mirror at scrawny pipestem arms and legs, caved-in chests, and feel like crying.

Because we live in a society in which almost half the population is overweight, someone who is very thin appears abnormal. But as long as the lack of fat isn't caused by a gross organic disorder, being underweight is often a distinct advantage! Underweight people live longer, suffer less from degenerative diseases and even psychiatric problems. In spite of their lack of bulk, they can (and often do) excel in sports that require specific skills like squash or track events.

They also look great in fashionable clothes. If you are thin but healthy, getting all the essential nutrients with plenty of protein, and if you are able to relax easily, then there is nothing to worry about, and you should count your blessings every time you see another article about dieting.

We are not really sure what causes excessive thinness, although there are a very few diseases where such a skin-and-bones appearance is a symptom. But they are really rare, and your doctor will check out any physical problem.

In some way, thin people are not good converters of carbohydrates – the body doesn't store it as much as it should, and you end up with a great deal of energy and no layer of fat. It is a fact that most thin people are also restless, highly-strung, and moving all the time. If you are healthy and thin, the chances are you will have to change your lifestyle to make any real change in your appearance. That means slowing down consciously, learning to relax, trying to make yourself do things carefully and gently, without whirling around like a dervish.

Although moderate exercise is always beneficial, your heart and lung capacity is likely to be pretty good. Spending an extra hour every day burning up calories is not really going to help. So settle for a brisk walk before meals as an appetite enhancer, and choose a sport that isn't particularly energetic. Swimming leisurely is one good choice, because it will also help to shape what fat you have into pleasantly lithe curves.

You may find suddenly you are starting to gain – usually it's because contentment and happiness have had their effect, and you are more relaxed and comfortable with yourself. Enjoy the new you.

HELPING TO GAIN WEIGHT

1. Try to make sure you are actually eating enough. Keep notes for a week or two – you may be missing lunch or dinner consistantly because you are too involved in your work or your family. If that's the case, regular meals, with a good assortment of nourishing dishes may well be the simple answer.
2. Learn to relax, and try to find a technique that suits you and the way you live. Try practising some form of relaxation before meals, even for five or ten minutes. Learn to take a deep breath every now and then during the day, and slow down.
3. Mild exercise will help tone muscles – they can be flabby and weak just as easily when you are thin.
4. Try to develop a real interest in food, exploring the different cultures, experimenting with new kinds of cooking techniques. Learn about wine, and serve it as often as you can – just a glass or two with dinner will somehow make you sit down and enjoy your meal and your surroundings.
5. Concentrate on eating one really good meal late in the day. Don't worry about breakfast too much – it will perk up your metabolism to even greater efficiency. Add carbohydrates if you can.
6. Have a good look at your life, and try to sort out some of the problems that might be causing you extra stress and strain. Get as much rest as you can, and try not to worry about unimportant things.

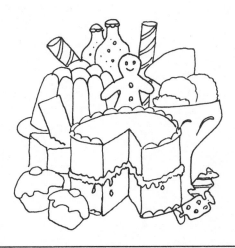

Diets For Children

YOUNG DIETERS

Perhaps the most important thing to remember about developing good eating habits is that children are as different and individual as everyone else in the family. Even the smallest toddler will have likes and dislikes, though the mother might think that all bland, pureed stuff tastes much the same. Don't assume that all children will gobble up a whole chocolate cake, and spit out even one leaf of spinach. If the attitude in the household towards food is relaxed and positive, with well-balanced meals that taste as good as they look, then children will grow up with a generally open mind. They'll be willing to try new dishes and unusual combinations, and if they eat a little more of one thing than another, it's not generally important. Nevertheless, there are times when children must be put on a special diet, because of illness or infection, or lovable plumpness that turns into downright fat. Different age groups have different problems, and have to be approached in slightly varied ways.

BABIES AND YOUNG CHILDREN

Young Children are easiest to deal with for the simple reason that nutritionally speaking, they are a captive audience, and almost always eat at home or with their parents. The best time to start solids, the best amount for your particular child, the formula you use and the quantity of milk are all the legitimate concern of the family doctor. It is not something you should pick up from friends or neighbors. Every child is different, and you are laying the foundation for a lifetime of good or bad health.

There used to be rigid schedules for every different theory, but today our whole attitude has become much more relaxed and adjustable. Nevertheless it doedn't mean anything goes! Find a medical adviser you can trust for advice, and also ask for a recommended book so that you can have a ready reference for small, day to day upsets or developments.

Young children begin to assert themselves as they become part of the family. Listen when when they express strong feelings about a particular fruit or vegetable and don't let it become an issue; then they won't learn to regard mealtimes as a battleground fought with 'good-for-you' vegetables against 'good-to-eat' desserts. Imagination plays a part, too, with appearance and associations rather than the taste – dark foods may be connected with night time and witches, whole sardines might seem to be almost alive, and so forth. When that happens, don't try to make them eat what frightens them. If you ignore the problem, it will usually go away. There are very few foods which cannot be replaced or sufficiently adapted to be acceptable.

Large servings of anything can discourage the appetite of a small stomach. Keep portions small and easy to handle – there are always second helpings. Attractive salads and garnishes help too, radish flowers and thin carrot sticks are fun and prettier for everyone and so are rolled sandwiches and star shaped cakes.

Don't get into the habit of disguising food all the time – all that does is develop a sense of perpetual fuss and special treatment which can be a problem later on.

Try and keep to the same nutritional standards for everyone – children burn up carbohydrates more easily than adults, but a fat child is *not* a healthy child, and when a youngster is constantly fed too much carbohydrate and fatty foods, cells actually develop differently, and all its life there will be a tendency to put on weight unless special care is taken. Growing children also need a higher proportion of proteins and vitamins and minerals.

CHILDREN AND SPECIAL DIETS

A child on an unnusual diet may have the psychological problem of feeling strange. Obviously with something like an allergy to protein or the inability to digest carbohydrates, or a form of diabetes, all food must be carefully watched. It's best to explain as simply as possible to the child what the diet is for. Explain that you won't be there all the time to check and he should learn to say 'I'm so sorry, I can't eat that,' or 'It will make me ill,' to foods he cannot eat. Encouraging the child to be specific also stops adults pressing the child to take something because they think it is politeness rather than real refusal. Make sure teachers know about the problem; they can keep an unobtrusive eye on shared treats or casual offers. Packed lunches for school, and allowable snacks to put in the pocket for playtime will help to keep a normal social life possible.

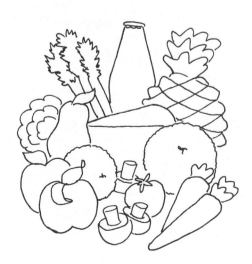

TEENAGERS AND SPECIAL DIETS

If there is a medical diet necessary to maintain good health, the young adult is usually capable of understanding what causes the problem, and avoiding the wrong food without too much difficulty.

Adolescence is the age when overweight may become a problem, especially with girls. Until very recently, it was an accepted 'fact' that older girls become less interested in sports, less active generally, quieter and more passive and mentally creative, rather than physically energetic. All this tended to burn up less calories, slow down the metabolism, and put on the pounds. In addition, natural hormone changes lay down protective cushions of fat on breasts, thighs and hips to make the distinctive rounded outline of the average sexually mature woman. Girls become more aware of their femininity, especially with regard to dress and fashion, and the current ideals of beauty which saturate newspapers, magazines and television. The vigorous, energetic 12-year-old slows down at 14, gains weight, and in a vicious cycle starts worrying about being fat. Even the appalling extreme of anexoria nervosa might result, however a more common result is an overweight teenager who needs reassurance and acceptance from friends, just as she looks or thinks she looks her worst.

Make sure that you both have the right attitude towards overweight. Thinness is not a virtue in itself, and fatness is not a punishment for sin. There are two valid reasons for losing weight, and by far the most important is the bad effect extra pounds have on your health. The second is psychological – you must be at home and comfortable with your own physical self, appreciate and enjoy your body, and treat it with care and affection. Together these two attitudes can transform your life, and your child's future, too.

Start with a good check-up at the doctors, to make sure there really isn't another problem. Family eating habits have a large part to play, of course, and statistics prove that one, or both, of the parents as well as the child would probably benefit from a better, more balanced diet. That might solve the problem gradually, without too much fuss, especially if it's only a matter of five or ten pounds.

Encouragement to join in exercises and sports with everbody else is an absolute must. 'Join in' is the operative phrase – if you expect her to be out there slogging away on the tennis court while you sit in a hammock, then don't be surprised if it becomes another losing battle – teenagers are very logical. Do as I do is a hundred times more effective than do as I say. It also stops her from feeling she is behind the great shame barrier – knowing that you are learning that keeping fit is vital for yourself, too, it won't be so lonely for either of you.

Make your whole approach into a positive companionship. If you think you'd benefit by losing a few pounds, so much the better. Didn't you always mean to try jogging every morning? Now's the time to try, no matter how busy you are. Or just experiment with a new kind of cooking or nutritional plan.

Sympathize with each other's problems, and treat it like a mutual benefit society. Involve her in meal planning, complete with calorie counts and lists of 'no' foods and 'yes' foods, but also involve her in the fun part – learning to cook new Chinese dishes with low calories and beautiful presentation, inventing new recipes, clipping ideas out of magazines. Of course, you will have had your doctor's advice about how much she needs to lose, and if her diet is stricter than yours, keep that fact as unobtrusive as possible. Encouragement and constant praise help a great deal, always with the right end in view – a better deal for herself. Remind her how much fun it will be to get into a marathon race or go skiing next winter. Find some activity she really wants to do, and encourage her as much as you can. Don't be too hard on the occasional lapse at a party,

and especially not in public – make sure she acts as your mentor, too; ask for encouragement for yourself, reminders to do *your* exercise, warnings before *you* go you to dinner.

And if for some reason you are exactly the right weight and unbelievably fit, then find something! You always thought it would be nice to be a black belt in judo, or an elderly Olga Korbut. And try for it! You never know – what may start out as a white lie may end up a burning ambition.

Don't forget the boys, either. Because most girls are more conscious of their weight, we tend to forget the quiet studious male roly-poly growing up beside her. Everything we've said can be read with him instead of her.

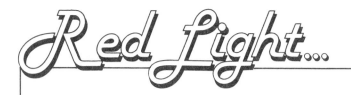

WHEN SHOULD YOU STOP?

In spite of everything we have said about the dangers of being overweight, there is a point at which trying to match some mental image of health and beauty can be downright dangerous. In a minor way, this kind of dieting obsession shows itself in compulsive worry; we all know the man or woman who is continually talking about food, trying out new diets, alternating between starvation one day and stuffing the next. A pound or two comes off, then one chocolate ice cream day, and it's all back again, until the next week.

From the health standpoint, an overweight person who see-saws back and forth puts more strain on the system than someone who stays slightly overweight.

But there's a far more serious problem that used to be very rare, and is now unfortunately becoming more and more common; a girl becomes so convinced that she is horribly, *obscenely*, fat that she stops eating, and if she is left without treatment, she may actually starve to death.

The condition is called anorexia nervosa, and it is mostly found among young, unmarried women, especially teenagers, although older women and men are affected every now and then. It often seems to begin with a normal interest in dieting, on the surface because the girl actually does need to lose a little weight, or simply because it is more fashionable to be as thin as a model. As the pounds drop off, she feels so successful and so virtuous that she doesn't want to stop.

By this time, she has become accustomed to eating so little that it isn't necessary to control her appetite – on the contrary, it becomes more and more difficult to eat at all. Food becomes the enemy, disgusting and degrading, and if worried parents and friends try to make her swallow she learns to pretend, and spits it out afterwards.

Endocrine disorders develop, her menstrual periods stop, her breasts become flat and child-like, and in fact her whole body reverses the normal process of growing up, and she becomes like a child again.

Even then, she seems unable to stop, and unless treated, she may continue to starve herself until it's too late and the body stops functioning altogether.

No one knows exactly what causes this kind of obsessive dieting. Some researchers have discovered a possible connection with a hormone inbalance, but most doctors believe that it is a sign of psychological problems.

Many girls seem to resent having to grow up, especially when there are family difficulties and rivalries which upset their lives. The patient wants to go back to childhood where it was safe and comfortable, without worrying about changes in her body, without having to cope with sexual feelings and the fear of pregnancy. She becomes again the dependent, helpless child, she has her mother's attention all the time – indeed, anorexia is *the* supreme attention getting device, and a very dangerous one. Even death becomes part of the game, a kind of 'you'll be sorry when I'm dead' gamble

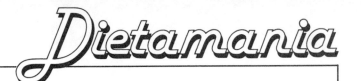

which doesn't always end happily.

Treatment is absolutely imperative, and very difficult; pleading or bribing is unlikely to have any effect, and professional help can take months or even years to be effective.

Usually the girl must be taken into hospital, away from the emotional atmosphere that has made her condition worse; by this time the frantic parents are themselves nervous wrecks as they watch their lovely, normal daughter turn into a walking concentration-camp victim.

Some kind of medical nutrition must be given, at least enough to help the body return to a normal state, even though the girl is still unbelievably thin. Once the body begins to work again, the real treatment can begin. And that means trying to find out somehow what caused the problem, and helping the girl to cope with her difficulties in a better way.

There are strange side effects, too; often the patient feels superior to other human beings because she can show such self-control, and if her feelings about being a woman were negative and 'unclean' then she will feel purified by denying the body so severely. Many seem to see themselves in a very distorted way – they actually believe that they are grossly overweight, and *need* to diet.

Whatever the cause, treatment can take a long, long time, and the patient may have several relapses later when emotional or sexual problems reoccur. So although real anorexia doesn't occur too often, it is worth

keeping an eye on teenagers in particular when they want to lose weight. Be sure you all know the facts about good nutrition and how it can affect physical and mental health. And don't get carried away by the symbol of the skin-and-bone models who decorate our billboards and magazines. They are not the ideal of love and beauty which most of us should want to copy.

Family Fitness

Introduction

FITNESS AND FUN

Don't be misled into thinking fitness is just being the right weight – an equation which means so much weight at so much height equals 'fit'. And if your scale gives the right answer, and whatever the weather you walk the dog every day, then the equation's perfect.

Sorry, there's more than that! Fitness is all about the state of your heart and lungs and seeing *they* get enough exercise, not just the dog. And that means you've got to do some sort of strenuous exercise regularly that actually leaves you breathless.

Going for a daily walk just isn't enough. It might make you feel good – and that's a good thing – but unless you walk very briskly (and drag the dog too fast) you're not exercising your heart at all.

Inactivity is beginning to shorten our lives. Heart attacks, high blood pressure, ulcers are all too common because we no longer use our bodies as they were designed. Now we barely move from place to place, except to step into our cars or hop onto a bus. Our bodies are actually deteriorating through lack of use.

It's a bit like leaving your car in the garage for months on end and then being surprised when it won't go. Just as your car works better when it's used regularly, so fit people's hearts are more resistant to stress, beat more slowly and are more protected against heart attacks and almost all known diseases.

So how can you tell if you're really fit? Try this simple test … experts reckon that if you're between 35 and 45 you should be able to complete a mile on the flat in ten minutes – in other words, travel at six miles an hour – without getting puffed and hold a normal conversation without gasping afterwards. Over 45 and you can add an extra minute for every five years. So at 50 you've got eleven minutes, 55 – 12 minutes and so on.

Another good guide is the state of your pulse which unlike blood pressure doesn't alter much with age. Run up two flights of stairs and it shouldn't really be more than 120 (that's beats per minute). If you don't know how to find your pulse, it's the thumb side of your wrist. Check it, by resting a finger there lightly and use a watch with a minute hand to count out the beats.

Not as fit as you thought? You can do quite a lot in your everyday life to improve things. Rearrange your day and walk to the station instead of driving … and walk briskly. Let the dog take *you* out rather than the other way round. And run upstairs as often as you can.

But while all these things help, they aren't the final answer. Regular exercise with deep breathing is the only way to keep your heart and lungs in good order. And this will involve some real physical effort. There's no easy way. Be suspicious if anyone offers you a short-cut – there's no substitute.

Nothing will make you fit overnight; fitness has to be worked at. You've got to build up slowly, doing a little more each day. Just ten minutes daily is better than hours once a week.

Sudden violent exercise does you more harm than good. It's a tragic fact that every year a few people collapse because they suddenly take up a sport or training programme after years of dog nothing. Doctors say anyone over 35 should have a check-up first, so should people with a history of heart trouble, back trouble or high blood pressure. And if you've recently had an operation, you should also see your doctor before attempting any sort of exercise.

Don't be too competitive either ... that's not what it's all about. There are lots of things you can do as a family. Get your children to accept sport and exercise as part of their daily life; it means you're equipping them well for the future ... and you can all have a lot of fun at the same time.

Just as important as the actual exercise is the relaxing afterwards. So many of us today suffer from tension – bringing on nervous headaches, stress pains at the back of the neck and shoulders.

It's worth learning the value of a little simple yoga, a warm bath plus massage. Deep breathing, as well as airing your lungs, will also help you to relax.

Our guide to fitness begins with exercises for all kinds of people – housebound mothers with only a few minutes, anxious teenagers who want to play in the school team, tired businessmen and women who need a break to get rid of the office tensions so they can enjoy an evening at home.

Then the sports, arranged alphabetically with groups for single people, then pairs, then a few team sports just to show you something of the range of possibilities.

Many of us just aren't any good at doing things unless there's someone there all the time to encourage us. That's the time to join a class where you'll be made to keep at it. If there's nothing in your area, get together with friends and neighbors and start your own.

There are television series which can get you off on the right track, or ask about records which have instruction booklets, music, and an encouraging voice to keep everybody bending and stretching.

Going to a health club is another solution but pick one that concentrates on fitness as opposed to figure shaping. There *is* a difference. Though any exercise is better than none, you want something to keep your heart and lungs ticking over nicely, not so likely at a beauty salon which is really intended only to help get your thighs trimmed down. Make sure they have exercise classes, too. Saunas and massage are wonderful for relaxation but you've got to earn it first.

Most of all, our message is a simple one – enjoy yourself! It's not just a question of adding years to your life, it's putting extra life into those years. Then you'll see that fitness really can be fun.

HOW TO BEGIN

So now you're convinced – you're even raring to go. Perhaps you woke up this morning and decided to run round the park or maybe you simply tried to touch your toes.

Good, it's a beginning. But don't rush at it, or you're less likely to keep it up. One good thing is that you're starting your routine for the right reasons. Most of us are drawn to exercising out of vanity. We don't like the shape of our bust or we think our thighs are too big. But the exercises we've devised for you put your heart and lungs first and cosmetic reasons last, with strength and mobility coming in between. It's really no good having a beautiful body if you can't run for the 8.10 train in the morning! It's nice to have both, though, and a really fit body is always a pleasure to look at.

Don't do too much, too soon. To begin with, you'll know if you're overdoing it if you feel very stiff. Don't do any more than we suggest at the beginning. As you get into shape you can begin to really strive for improvement. Then once it gets easy you can make it harder for yourself, but always stop if it's a real struggle.

Our series is for all the family but you must ease into it more slowly the older you are. Muscles are really like bits of elastic when they're in good condition and the longer you've left them unattended, the less stretchy they're going to be.

If you have any back trouble, (and over 40 %

of the population do) then be extra careful not to cause additional damage. Stop whenever it hurts – your own body is your best advisor. Never go on with anything that causes back pain.

The members of your family least likely to have any problems are the children, of course. They're generally fit anyway, though introducing them to regular exercise outside school will be equipping them well for the future. Any problems they do have will most likely be connected with posture.

If you're out of condition, at any age, or around the 40-year old mark, then take it easy, working up slowly to a *regular* exercise period each day. It's the continuous effort that counts.

On the opposite page are groups of exercises from this section. Choose a group that suits your age and your condition. As you become fitter, you can add extra exercises from other groups, one or two at a time. But remember to keep a balance so that all of your body gets some attention every time.

We start with a routine for beginners, or for older people just starting to get fit again. Choose four or five exercises for each week, changing them around to keep from getting bored.

1ST WEEK

SIDE BENDS	10
GOOD MORNINGS	5
SEATED STRETCH	5
FEET RAISERS	10
HALF SIT-UP	5
SIDE LEG RAISERS	8

2ND WEEK

SIDE BENDS	10
GOOD MORNINGS	5
SEATED STRETCH	5
FEET RAISERS	10
HALF SIT-UPS	5
CURL-UPS	10
SCISSORS	15
SIDE LEG RAISERS	10

3RD WEEK

SIDE BENDS	20
GOOD MORNINGS	10
SEATED STRETCH	10
FEET RAISERS	15
HALF SIT-UPS	8
CURL-UPS	15
SCISSORS	20
SIDE LEG RAISERS	15
HIP KICKS	15

4TH WEEK

SIDE BENDS	30
GOOD MORNINGS	15
SEATED STRETCH	15
FEET RAISERS	20
HALF SIT-UPS	10
CURL-UPS	20
SCISSORS	40
SIDE LEG RAISERS	20
HIP KICKS	20
SIMPLE PRESS UPS	10
SQUATS	5

5TH WEEK ON

SIDE BENDS	30
GOOD MORNINGS	15
SEATED STRETCH	15
FEET RAISERS	20
HALF SIT-UPS	10
CURL-UPS	20
SCISSORS	40
SQUATS	20
SIDE BENDS	30
GOOD MORNINGS	15
SEATED STRETCH	20
FEET RAISERS	25
HALF SIT-UPS	15
CURL-UPS	25
HIP KICKS	25
SIMPLE PRESS UPS	25

For those in good condition, who have already been doing some exercising. If it becomes too exhausting then slow down, and do fewer of each, but try to do at least 4 or 5 exercises every day.

	1ST WEEK	2ND WEEK	3RD WEEK
SIDE BENDS	30	50	50
GOOD MORNINGS	15	20	20
SEATED STRETCH	15	20	20
FEET RAISERS	20	2×20	3×20
HALF SIT-UPS	10	2×10	3×10
CURL-UPS	20	2×20	3×20
SCISSORS	40	2×50	3×50
SIDE LEG RAISERS	20	2×20	3×50
HIP KICKS	20	2×20	3×20
SIMPLE PRESS UPS	20	2×20	3×20
SQUATS	20	2×20	3×20

WARMING UP – four warm ups to get you going …

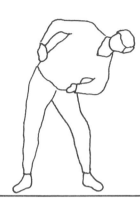
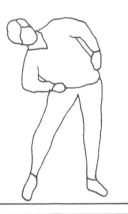

SIDEBENDS

A wonderful way to get your muscles warmed up. Start with feet wide astride and knees slightly bent. Then keeping hips as still as possible:
Bend to the right. Straighten up. Now do the same thing bending to the left. Work towards doing twenty each side.

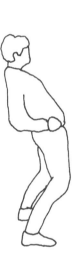
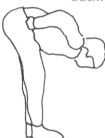

GOOD MORNINGS

Again start off with your feet astride and knees slightly bent. But this time bend forward, keeping your hips as still as possible. Straighten up and then arch backwards. Again aim at twenty.

SEATED STRETCH

As the name suggests start off sitting on the floor with legs as far astride as possible. Put your right hand on your left knee. Now try to touch your toes with your left hand and aim your nose at your knee. Swop sides and aim at ten a side. As you progress you can do three lots of ten.

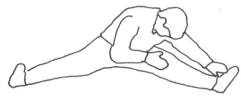
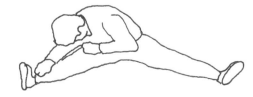

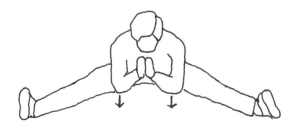

SPECIAL PELVIC STRENGTHENER
- this is a warm up exercise

You start sitting on the floor with your legs wide apart. Try to get your elbows down to the floor. Then with your arms outstretched try to reach as far forward as possible.

CURL-UPS
Start off lying down on your hands, with your head slightly raised off the ground. Now bring your knees up under your chin. Straighten legs out to an angle of 45 degrees and lower. Repeat twenty times.

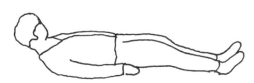

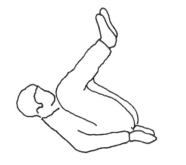

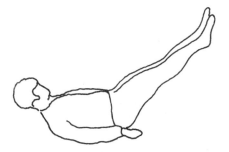

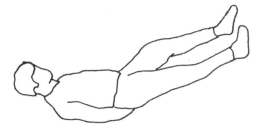

SCISSORS
Lie down with your legs at an angle of 20–30 degrees and your hands tucked under your bottom. Step Two – behave like a pair of scissors! Keep criss-crossing your legs. Work up to fifty.

135

HALF SIT-UPS

Start off with your knees slightly bent and your hands on thighs. Step two should have you sitting up to an angle of 45 degrees and trying not to move your legs and hips bringing your head to your chest. Again try for twenty.

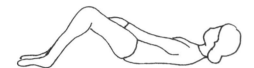

SIDE LEG RAISERS

Step one, lie on your side with your hand on the floor to balance you. Let your head resting on your other hand. Now lift your leg as high as you can. Repeat 20 times and then alternate with the other leg.

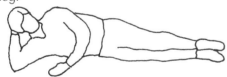

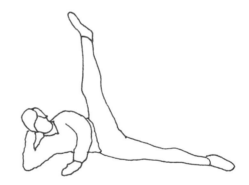

SIMPLE PRESS UPS

Start with your back straight and bottoms tucked in so that you make an unbroken line. Rest your palms on the table. Now lower yourself on to the table. You can toughen this one up by doing the same thing on the floor ... and later by raising your feet level as explained in our ten-minute fitness programme.

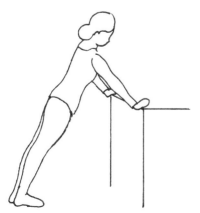

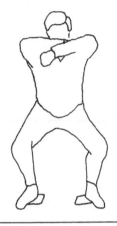
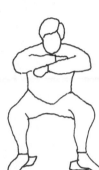

SQUATS

Start off with feet 15"–20" apart and also on a one or two inch block. Then keeping your back as straight as possible and your arms folded at shoulder level bend your knees to a full squatting position. Repeat twenty times.

PROBLEM AREAS

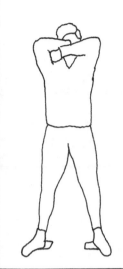

HYPER-EXTENSIONS (for Backs)

Lie down on your tummy with your feet tucked under a wardrobe. Now bring your body back as far as you can as illustrated. If there is any pain in your back or down the leg, stop.

... and to make it harder

Once you've really got the hang of this one try the same thing lying over a stool. Again bring your head and body back but make sure you choose a very stable stool! And you can make it even tougher by putting your hands behind your head.

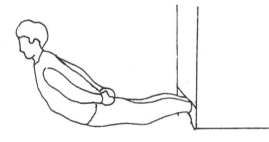

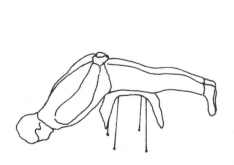

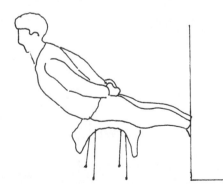

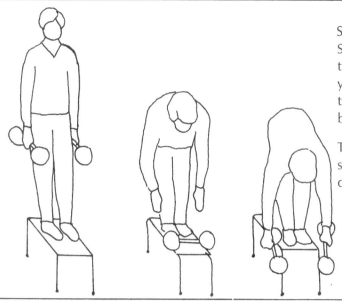

STIFF LEGGED DEADLIFT
Stand on a sturdy bench and, holding two weights, touch your toes. But when you get to your toes bend even further so the weights are below the level of the bench.

This is not advisable for anyone with the slightest back problem; it's basically for fit athletes only.

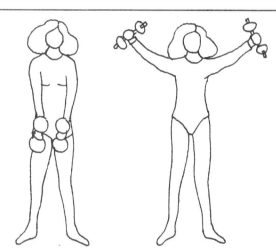

FLYERS (for busts)
You need your barbells or books. Feet should be apart and your hands at your sides. Take a deep breath and bring your arms upwards and backwards to just above shoulder level.

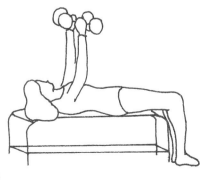

HIGH FLYERS (for busts)
Same as before but this time lie down on a bench with your 'weights'. Lower weights, keeping arms fairly straight, as low as you can.

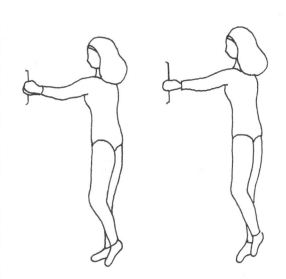

With holidays in mind ...

Still with the feminine interests at heart. If you're used to wearing heeled shoes and will be switching to flatties try this simple exercise ... it's also good for skiers, too.

FLEX FOOT GLORY
Find a firm step with something to hold on to nearby. Put your toes on the step and then your heels on the floor. Keep raising your feet. Repeat twenty times.

FEET RAISERS
Specially good for your tummy. Start off lying down with your hands under your bottom, palms downwards. Keep your head off the floor and legs completely straight with toes pointed. Now raise your legs up to an angle of no more than 45 degrees and then down again. Aim at doing twenty of these.

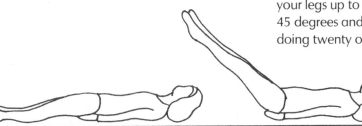

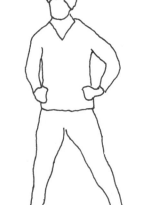

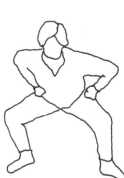

For knees and legs ...

DEEP KNEE BENDS
Excellent exercise for footballers. You start off with hands on hips, standing with your feet apart. Then lower yourself down, leaning forward slightly. Graduate to hands behind head, then to holding weights at shoulders.

LEG STRENGTHENER

Excellent exercise if you've been bedridden for a while. But it takes a little preparation. First you've got to have two weights for your feet … in a gym you would use special iron shoes. We tried it with a sturdy shopping bag with a few rocks from the garden or a few cans. Sit on the edge of the table with weight on or over foot. Straighten knee until leg is straight against resistance of weight. It is even better with the weight over your instep – point toes up, then straight, then point up again.

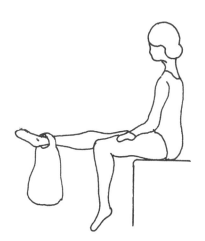

BREATHING BONUS (for stretching your rib cage)

Lie down on your back on a bench as picture. Take a deep breath. Lower the broom with straight arms down behind you. Recover to overhead position. Hold. Then repeat twenty times.

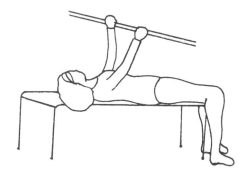

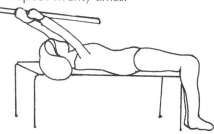

SITTING STRENGTHENER (for arms)

Start off sitting on a sturdy stool with your feet up on another one. Let your arms rest behind you. Now for the tough bit … try and sit down in the gap between the stools. Recover to straight arm position and repeat up to 20 times.

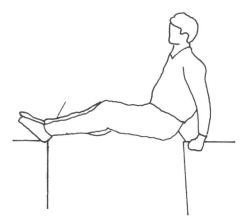

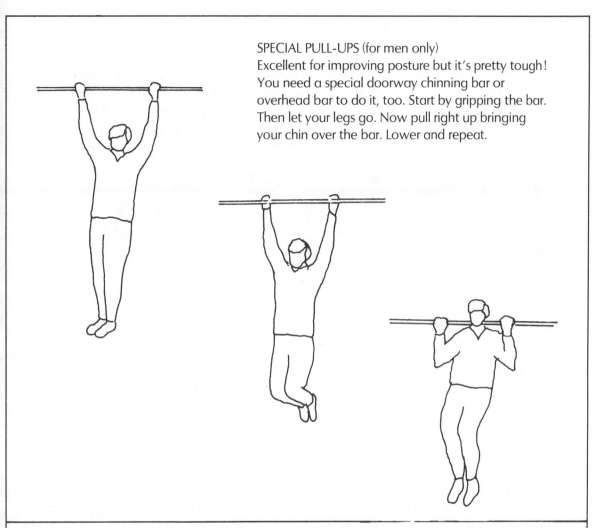

SPECIAL PULL-UPS (for men only)

Excellent for improving posture but it's pretty tough!
You need a special doorway chinning bar or
overhead bar to do it, too. Start by gripping the bar.
Then let your legs go. Now pull right up bringing
your chin over the bar. Lower and repeat.

WRIST ROLLER (for pianists, tennis players, cyclists, racing drivers)

Take a broomstick with a hole through the middle. Make sure the hole goes through diagonally. Thread rope through – see it's about four to five feet long – and tie it securely and then put a weight of about 5 lb at the other end. Hold at arms length and then run the handle round, keep winding the weight up. Your arms at shoulders' length and keep winding and unwinding for as long as you can. Five to ten times will suffice. You can use heavier weights later on.

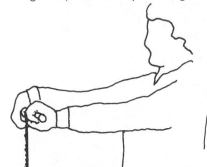

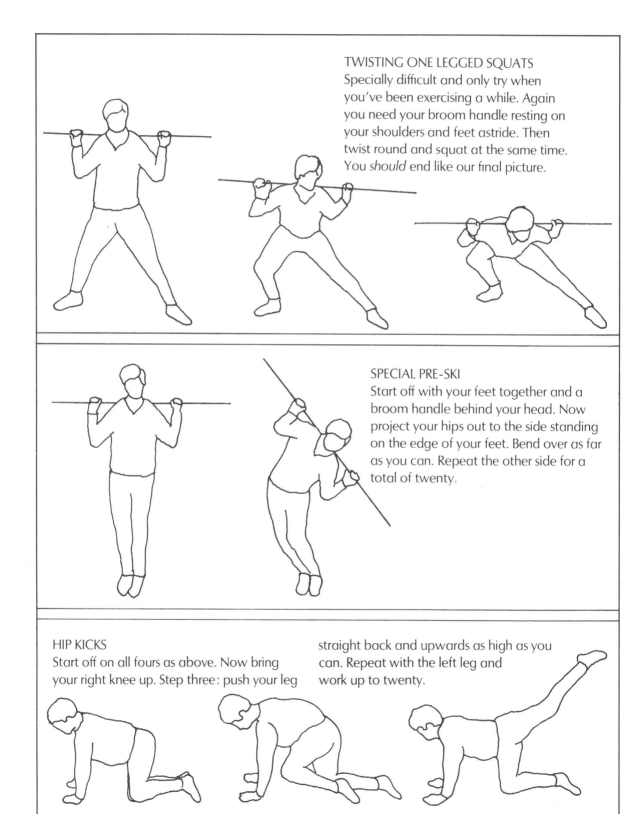

TWISTING ONE LEGGED SQUATS
Specially difficult and only try when you've been exercising a while. Again you need your broom handle resting on your shoulders and feet astride. Then twist round and squat at the same time. You *should* end like our final picture.

SPECIAL PRE-SKI
Start off with your feet together and a broom handle behind your head. Now project your hips out to the side standing on the edge of your feet. Bend over as far as you can. Repeat the other side for a total of twenty.

HIP KICKS
Start off on all fours as above. Now bring your right knee up. Step three: push your leg straight back and upwards as high as you can. Repeat with the left leg and work up to twenty.

SQUAT AND PRESS

One: So you can keep your balance you need to put your heels on a block about one to two inches. You need your 'weights' again, too. Hold them resting on your shoulders, elbows up.

Two: Keeping your back as flat as you can and your bottom slightly out as low as possible.

Three: Using your legs to 'drive' you recover to upright position pushing the weights overhead at the same time. Inhale as you sink back to squat position. Exhale when weights are overhead each time. Do these in sets of twenty.

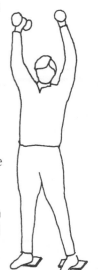

TWO HAND SWING

One: Hold something like small dumbells or a couple of books as shown. Start with your feet astride, holding your dumbells or books at arms length at waist level.

Two: Move your arms upwards to just above shoulder level, then lower bending your knees at the same time. From this bottom position thrust upwards with your legs so that those books swing right up above your head. Stretch for the ceiling.

Three: Now right down making a big arc almost to the floor before starting all over again. As you come back up see you 'drive' yourself with your legs.

Home Exercises

HOUSE AND GARDEN

Maybe you're the sort who just can't stick at a proper exercise routine. We're not blaming you but by doing no exercise at all you'll really be missing out. But all of us have chores to do so why not try combining the two? There are a host of things you can do as you tackle the housework or do the gardening ...

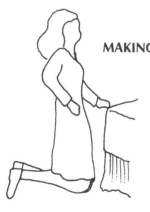

MAKING THE BED ... Think of your poor back and give it a break by seeing you always face the bed squarely. Try some deep knee bends while you work.

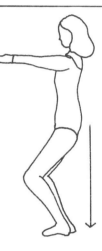

WASHING UP ... Do a few press ups against the sink top when you've finished the final pot. And more knee bends as you put them away in a low cupboard.

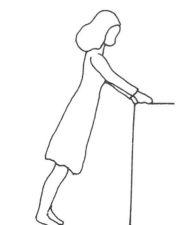

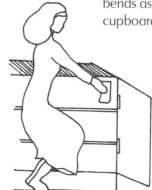

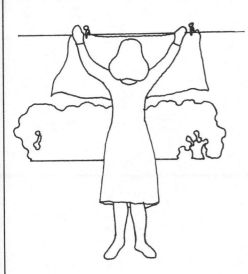

HANGING OUT THE WASHING ...

See the line high enough to force you into a good stretch ... and stretch over sideways each way before moving down the line.

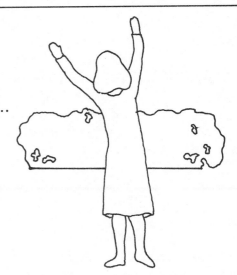

DUSTING ... Make sure your feather duster is short enough to force you to stretch up to shelves. Stretch-up is good for the youngsters, too. See you keep some of their toys high enough up so they really have to reach up for them.

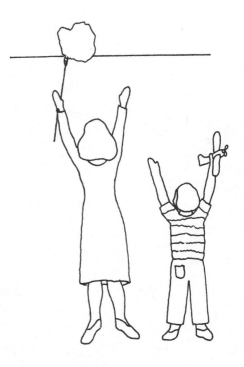

POLISHING ... Wonderful for firming up arms and bust – polish the furniture vigorously using each hand alternatively and making sure you get a good circular movement.

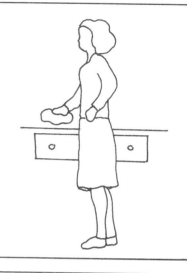

BROOM BONUS ... Four ways with a broom handle once the sweeping up is done.
Use the straight handle to twist from side to side, to help you pull into a sit-up, to add a lever to bending and stretching.

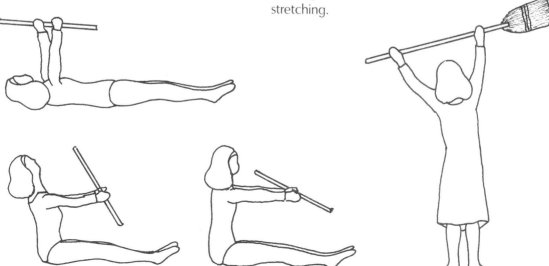

IN THE GARDEN ... Going mad in the garden is foolish – it makes you stiff for days and in extreme cases can be very dangerous. People have been known to have fatal heart attacks. Secret is to divide the work up – some weeding, digging, hoeing then weeding again.

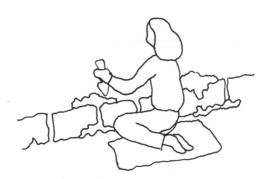

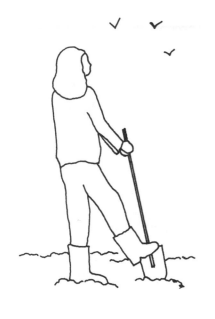

WEEDING ... Really get down to it by squatting for a while and then getting up slowly ... wonderful for thighs. Then switch to kneeling and make sure you've got a comfortable movable mat so you won't have to lean forward. You can try twisting from side to side provided you keep your back straight. See you slightly hollow your back as you kneel. Get up with a stretch.

DIGGING ... wonderful all over toner for arms, legs, and trunk but keep back as erect as possible and see you stop regularly to stretch up and back. Avoid bending forward.

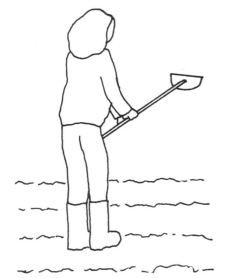

HOEING ... Don't overdo it and face the job straight. Stop every now and again for swings and knee bends ...

CUTTING THE HEDGE ... Using the shears firms bust and arms but make sure you relax afterwards by doing chest and arm stretches.

147

Isometrics

Isometric exercises are, by definition, the contracting of certain muscles by pressing any specific muscle against an immovable object so that when tension is applied, either by pushing or pulling the muscle does not expand or contract. The immovable object can be a wall, a heavy piece of furniture (heavy enough to withstand pressure of the legs, for example), or even another part of your body. Isometric exercises are used more for toning muscles rather than for body building.

Isometrics are useful to know because they can be practiced almost anywhere, at any time. When caught in a traffic jam, you can work on a few hand or arm pulls. If you're sitting at your desk at the office, you can do some leg presses. Even relaxing in front of the television, you can do the first exercise.

HEAD LOCKS

Lock your hands behind your head and press your head back as hard as you can. Hold the position for 15 seconds. Relax. Repeat five times.

This exercise will tone upper arm and neck muscles particularly. Place the palms of your hand against your forehead. Press forward as hard as you can. Hold for 15 seconds. Relax. Repeat five times.

Again this is excellent for toning neck muscles.

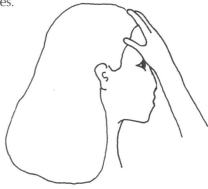

LIFT-OFF

With elbows bent and palms up, put your hands under the edge of a heavy desk or table. Flex your muscles as though you were trying to pick up the desk. Hold the position for 15 seconds. Relax. Repeat five times. This exercise is good for toning arm muscles, particularly the upper arms.

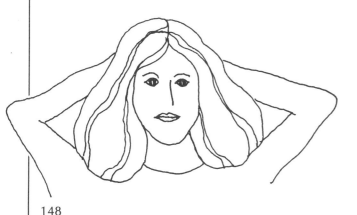

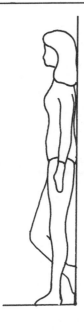

FRAME

Stand in a door frame, resting your back against one side of the frame. Lift one leg and press your foot against the other side of the door frame. Hold for 15 seconds. Repeat five times. Then do the same with the other leg. This exercise is particularly good for the upper leg muscles.

ISOMETRIC LEG HOLD

Lying on the floor with arms at the sides, palms down, slowly lift both legs a foot off the floor. Hold the position for up to six seconds. Keep your legs straight. Release, then repeat five times, at least twice a day.

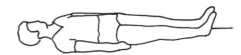

Look out! Although these exercises seem easy, isometrics can be an enormous strain on the heart and can raise blood pressure. If you have a heart condition or high blood pressure, check with your doctor before you begin.

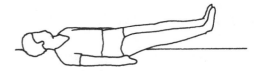

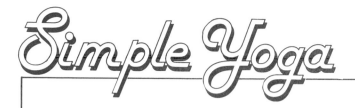

Simple Yoga

YOGA

Anyone can do it. You don't need a fantastic physique or to be amazingly fit. Although it is literally thousands of years old, yoga is especially good in helping to ease the tensions of the twentieth century. It's something the whole family can do too.

The word yoga means union and the philosophical ideal is to merge the individual spirit with the universal spirit, taking you on to a different level of thinking and feeling.

Many of the exercises are really quite simple and you can tackle the more complicated ones only when you are ready. A yoga session shouldn't leave you exhausted on the contrary! You should end up feeling wonderfully relaxed and filled with peaceful contentment.

There are three basic elements to yoga: the actual exercises or postures; the breathing, which is probably the hardest aspect to master; and finally, deep relaxation.

You should learn to make yoga a regular part of your daily life. Experts suggest that a few minutes every day is much better than one long session a week. Eventually, you should find practising yoga affects your whole lifestyle, so that you feel better all day, eat more sensibly, and as a bonus the deep-breathing exercises should even help you to give up smoking.

GETTING STARTED

Any loose comfortable shirt and trousers will do, but find a really comfortable rug or mat to lie on or you could end up bruising the back of your neck. You will find it much more instructive and more fun if you take a class.

BEFORE YOU BEGIN ...

● Anyone with a serious medical condition – especially high blood pressure, heart trouble or thyroid – should see their doctor first.

● Never practise on a full stomach – allow yourself a good two to three hours after a heavy meal.

● Although some aspects of yoga can be great pre-natal exercise, if you are pregnant consult your doctor.

● Don't let children start until they are at least seven and then only let them do the very simple things, because their bones and muscles are still not completely formed.

THE VITAL FIVE

Here is an exercise which you can do for five minutes, morning and evening, that will quickly retrain your breathing habits to make full use of your lungs:

Resting your hands on your rib-cage at the side, just above waist, breathe out completely. Now gently inhale through the nose letting your abdomen swell as much as it will to a slow count of five. Continue breathing in through the nose to another count of five, this time letting your ribs expand under your hands and finally your chest too (but don't raise your shoulders in the process). Hold your breath for a count of five. Now slowly let it out through your mouth counting to ten slowly, noticing how your rib-cage shrinks beneath your hands, and pulling in with your abdomen until you have released all the air. Do this five times in a row every morning and evening whenever you need an energy boost.

AND HERE'S HOW IT'S DONE ...

A selection of simple yoga exercises for all the family.

THE DEAD POSTURE

Not as dramatic as it sounds! Basically a relaxing position, it helps you recoup your lost energy at the end of a long, tiring day. So start and end your session this way. Lie as straight as possible, with your arms away from your body, feet apart as right and your palms upward. Don't fall asleep ... but it does help to keep your eyes closed.

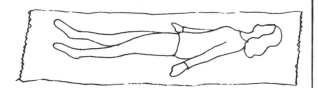

SITTING UP

Take it nice and easy. Inhale bring your arms up first with your fingertips erect. Then lower them slowly to your thighs. Raise your head, moving your hands at the last minute to your knees as you reach the sitting position. Hold, and then reverse slowly. Specially good for your spine.

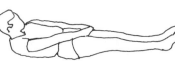
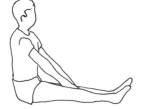

YOGA LEG RAISERS

Lie flat on the floor with your body completely straight. Now just inhale and raise one leg up after the other, holding for five to ten seconds. Exhale as you lower your leg. Do two rounds.

THE STAFF POSTURE

A good posture exercise. Sit with legs straight out in front of you and back completely upright and hands on floor as shown. But see you only balance on them, no leaning.

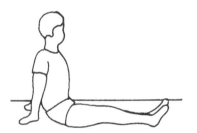

ADAMENT POSTURE

Good for the pelvic muscles and knees. Real enthusiasts claim it's helpful during menstrual cycle. Kneel down with your bottom in between feet. Inhale and raise hands over your head. Now exhale and come down on to your elbows as pictured.

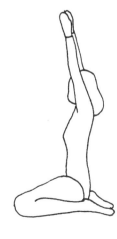

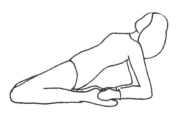

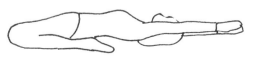

THE WINDMILL POSTURE

Basically a limbering exercise. Legs start apart, hands linked together in front. Bring them down then slowly round ... just like a windmill. Good for loosening the pelvis. Inhale as arms go up, breathe out as they come down. Three times each way.

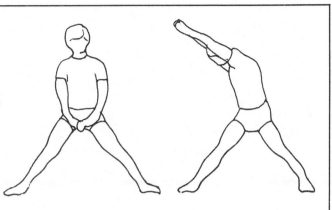

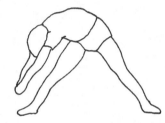 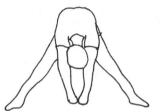

ALTERNATING KNEE TO FOREHEAD ... (WIND OF CHANGE)

This one is good for flatulence ... and consequently for reducing the weight around your stomach! Start off lying on the floor. Then take a deep breath and bring one knee up. Exhale as you bring your forehead to meet it. Repeat with the other leg and aim at three sets. Now try it with both knees up. As you breathe out, bring your head down to meet both knees. The third time try rocking when you're in this final position, getting as much movement as you can but don't touch the floor with head or feet.

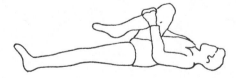 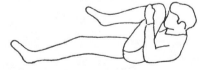

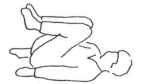 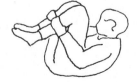

THE BUTTERFLY

Said to be good for thighs and flab …
and also an exercise pregnant ladies can
do but we'd advise you to check with
your doctor first. Sit down and literally
hold your feet in your lap as our picture
shows. Now let your legs flap … just like
a butterfly.

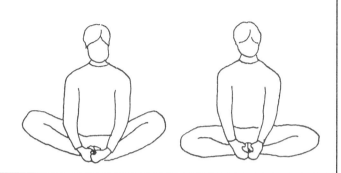

STANDING UP

If you're clever you can move straight into a
standing posture like the one right by
uncrossing your feet carefully. The standing
posture has your toes carefully lined up with
hands at right angles to your body.

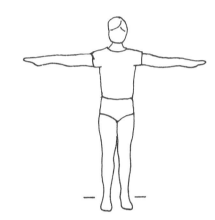

THE STRETCH

You'll find this one ideal for strengthening
ankles and legs. It also helps with poise and
balance. Take a deep breath as you bring
your arms up, then breathe out as you go
up on your toes. Inhale again as you stretch,
then as you bring feet down to the floor
breathe out.

Bring arms down to your sides and repeat
three times. Remember always to breathe
through your nose.

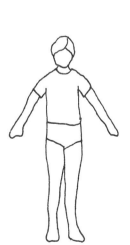
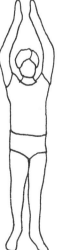
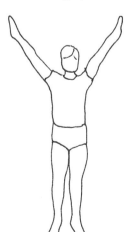
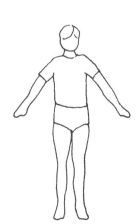

SHOULDER STRETCH

Feet apart, hands clasped behind your back. Stretch them right out as far as you can and drop your head back at the same time. If you're doing this one properly your mouth should drop open. Great for reducing tension in neck and jaw.

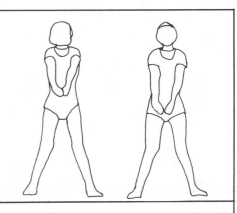

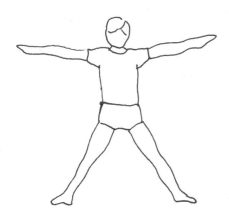

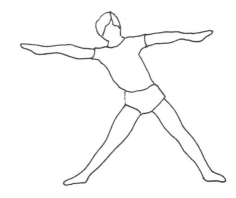

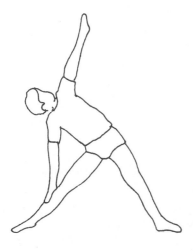

THE TRIANGLE

Start with arms and legs apart. Then inhale and lean over on one side. Exhale and slowly bring your hand down to your knee. Again too difficult for real beginners but something worth striving for. Do it to the right first and then the left.

During pregnancy, most fit healthy women should be able to continue with a moderate sport and exercise program provided the doctor approves.

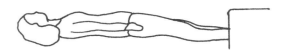

As the months go by and the baby becomes larger and heavier, very active sports become difficult and tiring, and eventually may be harmful. That's when exercises coupled with an intelligent and nourishing diet really comes into their own.

There are a few good basic exercises which are actually helpful in preparing for childbirth:

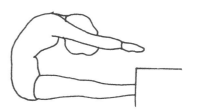

(1) Sit on the floor with legs as far apart as is comfortable. Put hands on your knees, then lean forward gently and relax until your head is as near the floor as you can get, let your hands slide towards your toes, and stretch down, bouncing lightly two or three times.

There are often complaints of backache when the last months are reached, so here is a simple back exercise to relieve the ache. It would be even better to exercise ten minutes a day before the backache begins!

(3) Lie on your back, knees bent, soles flat. Arms resting, press the hollow of your main back against the floor – hold for a slow count of four, then release. Breathe deeply, relax, then repeat.

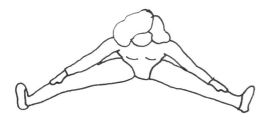

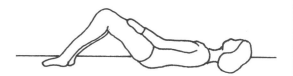

(2) Lie flat on your back, toes extended, tucked under a heavy chair or table. Bring your hands up, then pull yourself up to a sitting position gently and slowly.

After the baby is born, and the doctor approves, start exercising again gently to help the muscles get back to shape as quickly as possible. The longer you leave it, the longer the stretched skin will take to return to normal.

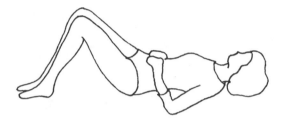

After the Baby...

But don't be foolish and hurt yourself. Begin with literally three or four minutes only – never do anything that hurts. If you get a cramp, stop at once and relax. Try something a little less strenuous the next day.

THE GREAT RELAXACISOR

Back Bend:
Stand with your feet a little apart. Knees straight, drop your head and let it get heavier and heavier, pulling your whole body into a curve, letting your hands fall free. Take a deep breath, hold it, and begin to pull yourself up uncurling your back like a cat. Still holding your breath, let the head drop back into the erect position, and slowly begin to breath normally again. The vital point is when you begin to uncurl, use your lower back muscles, do not pull your shoulders up.

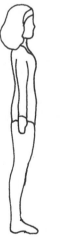
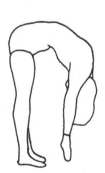

HOW TO GET YOUR FIGURE BACK …

It's what you've been dreaming about … being able to get back into closely fitting clothes after all those months of pregnancy.

And to help you get back into shape you'll need to exercise. But first check with your doctor and end each session with a period of relaxation.

The Day after the Baby – If your Doctor says Yes

(1) Great for toning up your tummy muscles. Start with your head on the pillow, knees bent and your feet flat as shown. Rest your hands about halfway down your tummy. Now breathe in deeply feeling your tummy go up. Then breathe out completely. Try to pull your tummy wall towards your back, in an attempt to squeeze out as much air as you can. Do this four times, three times a day.

(2) Toning up legs and circulation, another first day exercise. Lie down with your head on the pillow and legs straight out. Now bend and stretch ankles. Try pointing feet upwards. Keep your ankles as still as you can, then bend and stretch your toes. Circle your feet outwards, now do the same thing inwards. Repeat four times, three times a day.

(3) Stay lying down with your legs straight. Try pressing the backs of your knees and thighs downwards as hard as you can on to the bed. Relax. Four times, three times a day.

(4) Very important … an exercise for the pelvic muscles. Keep your head on the pillow but this time your knees bent and slightly apart. Feet should be flat. The best way to do this exercise is to imagine there's a piece of string attached halfway between your vagina and back-passage, running up through your body towards your chin. What you've got to try to do is tighten your muscles as if to pull up the string inside you. Do this as slowly as you can – the pressure should be inside, not around the hips and tummy. Now relax. Four times as before.

Three days after the birth you can add:
(5) With a trim waistline in view, start of as illustrated with one leg bent, keeping that still while you try to make the straight leg shorter by drawing it up from hip and waist. Then make it longer by stretching down instead. Repeat with the other leg up to four times once a day but after several days you could make this five.

(6) For your tummy … start off with knees bent and feet flat. Now tighten your tummy muscles and pull in. Press your waist downwards, as hard as you can to round spine. Keeping your waist in contact with your bed or the floor, lift hips off it slightly by contracting your bottom. Now relax. Up to four times once a day as before.

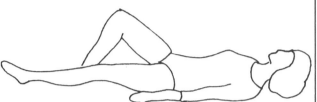

(7) Start off lying down with knees bent and arms stretched out at your sides. Twisting from the waist only, swing both knees to touch the bed on the left, then swing over to the right. See you keep your feet and shoulder still and knees firmly together. Excellent for waist and hips. Repeat as before.

Fourteen days after the birth you can add some more difficult ones … and don't use the pillow for these
(8) Start off as shown with arms at your side. Lift your head just a little and your shoulders, too. Bend to one side, reaching down with your arm. Repeat the other side.

(9) This time put your hands on the top part of your chest. While your waist and back ribs stay firmly on the floor, lift your head and shoulders up. Keep your eyes fixed on your bent knees. Now lower and relax. Specially good for your midriff.

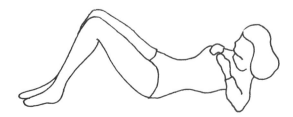

(10) Start off as before but hands at your sides. Now lift your head and shoulders a little and with your right hand touch the floor on your left side, all the movement coming from the waist. Repeat the other side.

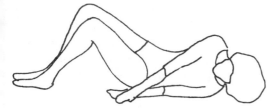

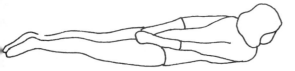

(11) Fold your arms under your head, as shown, letting your neck muscles relax. Lift each leg in turn; stretch gently, then relax.

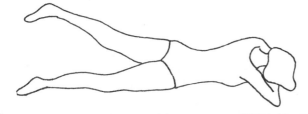

LATER IN LIFE

You can't start planning too soon for your later years. If you don't tackle your weight problem today, by middle age, not only will you find it harder to shed those extra pounds, but your skin will be so badly stretched that it may be nearly impossible to get yourself into truly good shape. Even more important, remember the old saying 'Use it or lose it'. This may be extreme, but you must make sure that *all* your muscles are exercised regularly or your chances of pushing them back into motion will be very poor.

Most of us worry about having sufficient money when we retire; people who don't make adequate financial plans are regarded as foolish. But too few of us think about making sure we'll be *fit* enough to enjoy our later years when they come. As we live longer and doctors learn how to cope with most major diseases, the time of life after 50 looks increasingly exciting. But your body needs to be fit in order to enjoy these years to the fullest.

If you are over 50 and have not exercised before, don't convince yourself that it is totally hopeless. *It isn't.* You must be sensible and get a thorough physical check-up first; that's all.

Explain to your doctor the type of exercising you plan to begin and ask him to provide any warnings he may deem necessary. For example, if you have such problems as heart disease or varicose veins, he may limit the time you spend exercising or caution you against certain types of exercises.

Always begin exercising moderately and establish a regular routine. (Sporadic exercise at any age is useless and can be quite dangerous to older people.) Keep at it! Before long, you'll be as active and fit as your children.

Most adults pride themselves in looking younger than they are. A few areas of the body are prime targets for the aging process: The face, the neck, the hands, the feet, and the back. Here are some tips to keep all of these crucial areas young and supple.

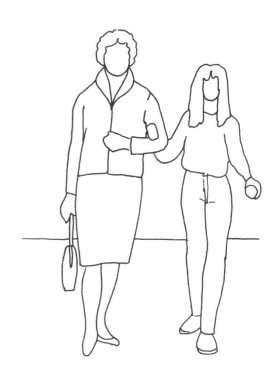

THINGS TO DO

NECK
Though some sweaters and scarves may hide a multitude of sins, strengthening the muscles that prevent the aging of the neck is a much better solution. Sit down to do this exercise or you may feel dizzy. Rotate your head from side to side, then tuck your chin in as far as you can, touching the breastbone as many times as you can.

FEET
To look after your feet, make sure that you have at least two pairs of shoes in regular daily use and when you're indoors, walk about without them on as much as you can. If you're overweight, your feet really do take the extra strain.

Put them back on the road to improvement by simply picking up a pencil with your toes a dozen times a day. Another good foot exercise you can do while watching TV is to rotate your feet at the ankles and bend them up and down. See p 224 for more.

BACK
Back trouble makes you feel terrible whatever age you are, but as you grow older, even more care is needed. Here are some tips worth remembering. Always let *both* legs take the strain. Many of us naturally put more weight on one or the other leg, so try consciously to correct this. Always keep your head up and your shoulders straight and the lower part of your back flat. If you're uncomfortable in your car, get a cushion to fit into the small of your back.

FACE
A sagging face makes you look old and makes you feel older, too. Here are three simple aids. Give a large yawn, opening your mouth as wide as you can. Try raising your eyebrows as high as you can, holding them up for a few seconds before lowering them. Next, close your eyes as tightly as possible, keeping them shut for as long as you can. Relax, and try again.

HANDS
To keep your hands limber and supple, practice these two simple exercises. First make as tight a fist as possible. Relax, then stretch out your thumb and fingers as far as you can. Don't forget to try both hands. Next hold out hand with fingers and thumb outstretched. Tense all the muscles as tight as you can while still outstretched.

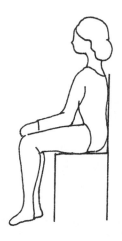
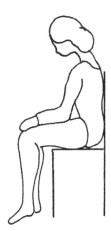

A Sporting Chance

BEING A GOOD SPORT

Look at the history of many sports, particularly the older ones, and you'll see that they began as skills needed for survival in a hostile and alien world. Javelin throwing and archery made Sunday's dinner possible, swimming took you across the river from the danger of bush fires or hunting animals, fencing kept your wits about you when attacked on all sides by warrior tribes.

In so many ways, life seems to come full cycle, and sports are no exception. We may not have to hunt or wrestle, but we do have to face up to other killers which are just as dangerous, and even harder to pin down. Heart and lung diseases, obesity and digestive illness are the modern version of horror stories for the middle-aged, and it's never too late to begin learning how to cope with them.

One note of warning: some sports will tend to make you arch your back, and if you have back trouble that will make it worse. Generally speaking if you feel the strain, take it easier. This applies particularly to strenuous movements – hard serves in tennis, a racing crawl stroke in swimming. But don't let taking it easy mean give up. It's quite clear that every day you stay fit and lively adds months and years to your life.

Remember that laughter and good spirits are as important as good physical health. That's where sports, especially group sports, really come into their own. Some are extremely good exercise and very efficient in using muscle power and burning up calories but they are also an enjoyable way to relax. Our calorie-burning counts are an average for the normal human being playing reasonably well.

Most sports have national organizations that provide rule books, and can guide you to local clubs. See the appendix for a listing of all organizations representing your favourite sport and write for further information.

Remember that this section is for families and enthusiastic beginners, to help you find something that might appeal to you as a way to enjoy yourself with the family and keep fit at the same time. So we have not attempted to cover professional sports or give too much technical information. The individual societies have booklets and advice when and if you want to become a better player.

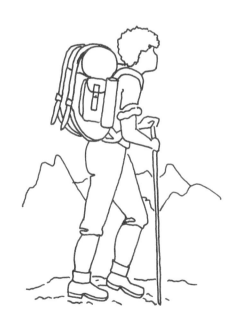

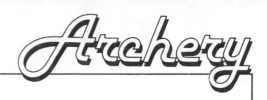

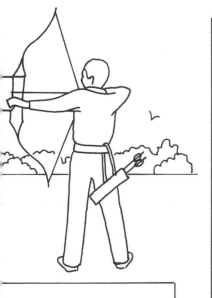

BOWS AND ARROWS

Archery may not seem very energetic, but it scores top marks for recreation, enjoyment, and co-ordination of hand and eye. Pulling back the string of a championship bow can take an effort of up to 42 pounds, even though it's not a high energy sport – about 30–40 calories in ten minutes. There's plenty of room for ambition – archery is a recognized, international and Olympic sport, with a governing body, competitions, and world championships. But it's also an exciting outdoor game for everyone, provided you remember that bows and arrows are still dangerous weapons to be treated with respect.

Popular target archery needs an open, fairly sheltered field with about 300 feet between the shooting line and the target, plus another 75 feet beyond as a safety zone. For beginners, the shooting line is nearer the target.

Wooden or composition bows are graded in pounds measuring the strength needed to pull the arrow back (men up to 42 pounds, women up to 34). Arrows are different sizes graded according to the height of the archer. The padded straw target is painted in circles; the gold bullseye rates ten, while the outer white ring scores only one.

Once you shoot reasonably well, there are all kinds of competitions and friendly matches – even light-hearted variations where archers and golfers match shot for shot around a golf course. Robin Hood and William Tell haven't faded away yet.

BEFORE YOU BEGIN

● There is no such thing as a toy bow and arrow. Even a child can let fly a careless, but fatal shot. Watch young children carefully, and learn the basic safety regulations.

● If you are interested in field sports, try Field Archery instead of Target Archery. They shoot over rough ground at different targets.

WHAT YOU NEED, WHERE TO GO, HOW TO LEARN

● No special dress is required, but simple sport clothes and comfortable, flat-soled shoes are best.

● You must have a special glove on the pulling hand, and a leather bracer on the other forearm to protect you from the rebounding string. Some clubs have old ones for beginners.

● Bows and arrows can usually be rented for the first few lessons, but practice bows are not expensive. You'll also need to hire a quiver for the arrows. Bring a cloth or towel to wipe dirty arrows.

● Learn to shoot by joining a local club or society, or find a qualified coach.

● Never try to learn by yourself, and **NEVER** practice on an unprotected stretch of ground.

Ballet and Dance

ON YOUR TOES

Classical ballet began in 17th century France when folk dances were stylized for presentation at court. In the 19th century, *corps de ballet* were trained to appear in European operas. For many years, the Russians kept up a strong classical dance tradition in the French form, and dancers use the French vocabulary for all ballet steps.

There are a number of steps and movements which begin from the five basic positions and most teachers follow traditional methods which join arm and leg movements in graceful sequence.

Modern dance is not simply a form of ballet, it is a total break from the classical ballet tradition. Modern dance grew up in America through the efforts of Isadora Duncan, Ruth St. Denis, Martha Graham, and many others. Today, it is one of the most popular arts, and many of the movements and routines add interest and fun to exercise classes, keep-fit clubs and children's physical education lessons.

Both ballet and modern dance are fun as well as being graceful and interesting ways to keep fit. People who find plain exercise boring should try taking an introductory dance class. The warm-up exercises which, for the most part, are standard in both ballet and modern dance, are simple to do, but they limber up all your muscles. You have the added pleasure of exercising to music and the added challenge of learning dance techniques.

WORTH NOTING

Dancing is the perfect all-round exercise. Classes are designed to stretch and develop every muscle in the body; feet, legs, back, pelvis, hands, arms – even the face. Most classes are divided into three parts; warm-up exercises, technique on the floor or at the barre, and floor work.

WHAT YOU NEED, WHERE TO GO, HOW TO LEARN

- For all kinds of dancing, a leotard and tights are really the best clothes to wear. A sweatshirt or sw to put on after class is a good way of keeping muscles warm.
- Ballet shoes: soft leather slippers for beginners of all kind, romantic pink satin toe shoes only when teacher allows it. Many shoe shops stock the slippers; you'll need a specialist for the toe shoes.

- You must begin in a class. Look in the telephone directory for local schools, write to your national organization, ask at schools and health clubs. Most beginners' classes are not expensive but remembe you'll need to go regularly to get the full benefit.

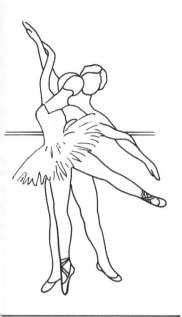

MOTHER AND DAUGHTER

Although dancing is something for both sexes, it is mostly women who attend classes, so it's good to remember that young girls benefit as much as their mothers. All forms of dancing are good for posture and balance.

GETTING STARTED

For exercise and fitness, whether you take ballet or modern dance classes is purely a matter of personal preference – ballet is based on a precise set of movements with a strong traditional background. You'll need flexible ankles if you hope to progress to wearing toe-shoes.

Modern dance is much more informal, and there are various teachers and schools with very different techniques and methods of instruction. Physically it's a lot easier for the beginner, since there is no toe-work, and your size and shape aren't so important.

Of course, as you improve, so does your stamina and suppleness, and it becomes really exciting to see the change in your posture, and overall vitality.

You should always begin in a class, since both kinds of dancing can lead to muscle strains and injury unless you get qualified coaching. It is quite strenuous, and most classes will work you very hard for one or two hours, burning up around 120 calories in ten minutes.

Once you are started, you can practice at home but even the best professional dancers take classes regularly.
If you've been really out of condition, or you are middle aged, then it's good idea to go to your doctor before you begin a tough course of lessons, but once you are fit again, you can go on dancing for a long, long time.

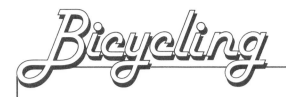

Bicycling

WHEELS FOR EVERYONE

Not just a sport, a bicycle can be useful as a form of cheap transport. More and more people have found buying a bike pays for itself in less than six months and also provides a practical way to get their exercise.

Children love bikes too, and outings for everyone in the family are wonderful ways of getting to know your area, and all the local beauty spots.

Using your bike regularly will do you *and* your heart and lungs a lot of good. Cycling gets top marks for promoting endurance, muscle development and co-ordination, plus a good return for all the energy you put in. Travelling 15 miles an hour, you will burn up 115 calories in just ten minutes. Some heart specialists recommend cycling for cardiac cases although anyone in this situation must always check. Cycling can also be a competitive sport; there are a host of activities available, everything from long rallies which can last days or even weeks to short sprints around an indoor track. Stay-at-homes could try an exercise bicycle to pedal away in the privacy of their own room, but you won't get anything like the fun of spinning along in the fresh air.

WORTH NOTING

Never attempt to ride on a main road till you're really confident. Even then, cycling in towns and cities can be hazardous. Try to find paths set aside for cyclists only.

OLD TIMERS

The original boneshaker came on the scene in 1865. Today, collecting and restoring old bicycles can be a special bonus. Prints and illustrations of changing cycle fads and fashions are good finds — bike to secondhand bookstores and antique dealers.

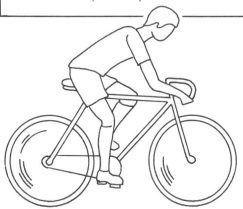

A CHILD'S BIKE

Buying a bike for a child needs great care, and it's as well to seek expert advice. The weight and the size are especially important. Don't let 'he'll grow into it' be your guide – a child trying to cope with a bike he can't handle is a danger to himself and others.

WHAT YOU NEED, WHERE TO GO, HOW TO LEARN

- Apart from the bike, you need close fitting shoes. Leather soles are better than rubber.

- Wear tight fitting trousers or clip them at the ankle.

- You'll need a good pair of gloves for cold weather. Leather ski gloves are ideal. A cap and cape are needed for when it's wet.

- Practice makes perfect. Find a traffic-free place, take a friend to cheer you along and keep on trying!

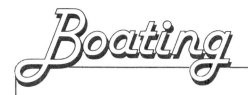

Boating

CANOEING KAYAKING AND ROWING

The traditional canoe is long, not too narrow, solid enough to carry loads for camping trips. Most hold two or three people comfortably, kneeling in the open shell and using a longish paddle. A kayak is generally smaller, perhaps 18 feet long, and the top is covered in. One or two holes let the paddlers climb in and sit down, and they use a shorter, double-bladed paddle.

The familiar rowboat is much more stable, with a longish oar attached to a pivot on the side. Racing boats are specially built and are usually available only to clubs – they have long oars carried by suspended riggers two or three feet from the boat itself.

There are competitions for teams and amateur associations, with long-distance racing and slaloming classes for canoes and kayaks. Slalom has been adapted from skiing, and it's dangerous and exciting, with contestants speeding down stretches of very rough water through numbered gates.

There are quieter ways of enjoying boating, and it's first-class exercise; canoeing and kayaking can burn up 100 calories in ten minutes, more if you're racing. Rowing is a bit more leisurely – only 45 calories for the same time.

A bonus is being able to enjoy the changing waterside, and modern canoes are so light they can be picked up easily and carried home if your stream runs dry.

WORTH NOTING

- All boating sports are only for those who can swim; always wear a life jacket, especially if you are with a small group.

- Take a waterproof bag with a towel and change of clothes.

- Never go out alone unless there are other people within easy distance. Don't explore by yourself, particularly in rough water and coastal areas.

- Tell someone where you are going, and when you intend to be back.

- Remember large canoes can take up to four or five people for family trips.

WHAT YOU NEED, WHERE TO GO, HOW TO LEARN

- No special clothing is needed; comfortable trousers and a shirt will do nicely in warm weather. In winter, you'll need extra sweaters, and perhaps even a wet-suit when it's really cold.

- Light, flat-soled shoes are best; tennis shoes are ideal.

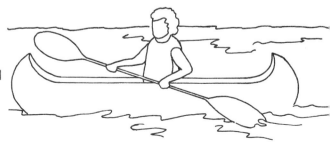

Body Building

MUSCLE POWER

Forget the strong man at the circus in the leopard skin. That's just not what modern body building is all about. Probably more than any other sport, body building has misconceptions about it – such as, you have to be born big, strong – and dumb – in order to participate. In fact, body building really demands a well-developed knowledge of the human body. It has recently enjoyed a tremendous surge in popularity even with women, who are interested in developing the perfect figure.

Body building is precisely what its name implies – a scientific working up of every muscle in the body. A number of exercises using various types of equipment – each with a precise purpose – are prescribed. As with dance and gymnastics, you should always begin body building with proper instruction or muscle malformation or injury can result. In addition, you should plan (or have an instructor plan for you) a specific exercise routine, and you should exercise at the gym at least twice a week.

Body building is very strenuous. If you are over forty, you should have a check-up with your doctor before you begin. Because the equipment is somewhat complicated and requires strength, this is not a good sport for young children; although it might be perfect for adolescents, especially those who are self-conscious about their bodies.

BEFORE YOU BEGIN

● Make sure you have a qualified instructor before you begin any kind of work out.

● Always do a few warm up exercises (sit ups, bounces, or jumping jacks etc.) before you begin. Your muscles must be warm or you can injure yourself.

WHAT YOU NEED, WHERE TO GO, HOW TO LEARN

● You should wear a sweat shirt and shorts. A leotard would be suitable for women. Non-slip gym shoes are required.

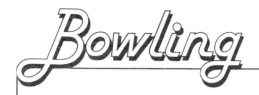

Bowling

BOWLING ALLEYS

Bowling couldn't have a more modern image, but a stone ball and nine pins were found in the tomb of a child buried in 5200 BC. So it has been around for centuries. All that's really happened is that the simple concept of throwing a ball at a target has become a lot more sophisticated.

This is fast, exciting and highly competitive sport, played in specially built bowling alleys of any number of wooden, highly polished lanes 60 ft long. A group uses one lane, and the players can compete against each other, or as a team against another group. The balls are very heavy, and quite large (about $13^1/_2$ inches diameter) with three holes to give a grip. Each player rolls his ball in turn down the lane, towards ten wooden pins standing in place at the other end. The score's based on knocking down the most pins with as few balls as possible. There used to be ball boys running out to put up the pins each time, now it's all done by machine.

The balls can vary in weight and you pick one to suit yourself. What you should try for is a strike, knocking down all the pins at once. For this you get ten points plus the score of the next two balls bowled.

One of the greatest assets of bowling is the social atmosphere. The alleys are noisy, usually crowded, with plenty of players and spectators of all ages watching and waiting for their turn. Friends play together, or in clubs; everyone can join because it's not too difficult.

WHAT YOU NEED, WHERE TO GO, HOW TO LEARN

BOWLS:

● A set of four bowls, usually called woods although they may be made of composition as well. Find out if a local club has sets to hire, as they can be quite expensive to buy.

● Join a club by writing to the national organization, or go along to the green and see if you can join a team.

● Get a willing expert to give you a few pointers, then just play. You can practice at home, too, even on not-too-perfect lawns, and the family can make up your team.

WHAT YOU NEED, WHERE TO GO, HOW TO LEARN

● Wear professional shoes, which can usually be rented at the alley. Otherwise, tennis shoes are usefu

● Comfortable casual clothes – no tight sleeves.

● Most areas have a bowling alley nearby. They often get crowded in the evenings and at weekends, you have to book a time; call before you go.

● Learn by playing, preferably with someone who plays regularly. Ask at the alley about local teams – many clubs have regular bowling nights. But it's a real family sport, inexpensive, fun.

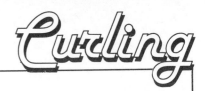

Curling

CURLING:

● Warm, well-fitting gloves, comfortable, warm clothes. Some players prefer shoes that slide, others use rubber soles.

● Stones can usually be hired from a club or at a rink. They are very expensive to buy, but a well-made pair would probably last you a lifetime.

● Learn by watching and practising. Check with your national organization or ask at the rink about joining a local team.

OUTDOOR BOWLS

Sir Francis Drake finished his game of boules before sailing off to defeat the Spanish Armada, and three thousand miles away the tip of Manhattan Island is called Bowling Green. So bowls are a part of history. Old fashioned, perhaps, but relaxing, mild exercise.

The Green is a lawn about 40 yards square, divided into six lanes, or rinks. You can play against each other, or in teams of two to four. Each player in turn rolls a ball down the rink, trying to get nearest to a small white ball, the jack.

There are indoor greens in some areas, made of synthetic grass. They help to make bowls a game for all the year round. Bowls are particularly adaptable for the blind or disabled.

CURLING

A kind of stone bowls on ice, curling is played in almost every northern country. Traditionally it began in Scotland where burly highlanders hurled 100-pound boulders down frozen rivers and lakes, but indoor rinks have encouraged everyone else to join in. In Canada it is almost a national occupation.

The modern curler needs skill as well as strength. The rounded granite stones, about 44 lbs, are slid from one circle cut in the ice to another, around 40 yards away.

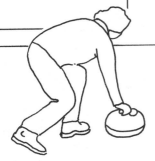

SPECIAL NOTE:

All kinds of bowling are especially good as you get older. They don't burn up too much energy – about 70 calories in ten minutes play – but they encourage supple muscles and the bending and stretching is first-class exercise.

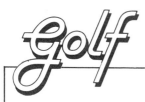

ABOVE PAR

It is said that Mary Queen of Scots enjoyed a game now and then; by the time she reigned, golf was already a Scottish national pastime. In 1457 Parliament banned the game because too many men were abandoning their archery practice and rushing off to play golf. A habit many present day golfers would appreciate.

What is it that has captured so many people from so many different parts of the world? Partly it's the versatility; golf is played against a score-card rather than against other competitors, so you are really playing against yourself. For the family, that means that everyone can enjoy playing together, even if one is an expert and one a complete duffer. A handicap system means they can all have a good match.

Then, too, it isn't physically very demanding, using up only 50 calories in ten minutes play. Older men who might not feel up to a hard tennis match can still play 18 holes of golf. Golf courses in milder climates are open all year; they will close only for heavy snow and ice. And for the closed period, or when heavy rain drives the players away, there are driving ranges and even indoor schools to practice individual strokes. Putting greens can be mocked up on a bit of flat lawn, or even on a square of carpet, so you can practice at home.

Finally, golf is one of those rare games where the absolute beginner can play like an angel, and the star of the club can have a disastrous round. It's a game of luck, as well as skill, and the next day may just be yours.

GOLFING MANNERS

Golf can be dangerous – the ball travels at very high speed. Players can be hidden by trees or hazards, so check carefully that there is no one ahead of you within hitting distance when you play. There are many regulations about etiquette – letting other players through, replacing divots when your club has lifted a section of turf, and so on.

WHAT YOU NEED, WHERE TO GO, HOW TO LEARN

- Comfortable casual clothes are all you need, a knit shirt is useful so you can swing properly. Golf sho have spikes to grip the ground but any kind of comfortable walking shoe with rubber soles will do. Golf gloves are useful to prevent blisters.

- Clubs and courses usually have a shop run by the professional coach, called the pro shop. You'll be able to rent clubs there, and probably get a couple of used balls for your first round.

- Ask at the pro shop about lessons, first . A few lessons are really worth while, and there are indoor g schools, too. Then book a time to play at the course, and turn up on time or you'll lose your place.

- Driving ranges are places to go and practice long shots; you can usually rent a club and a few buck or balls.

GETTING STARTED

Basically golf is a ball-and-club game involving two skills, propelling a small, hard ball in the air for anywhere from 30 to 600 yards, then putting the same ball on the grass into a tiny hole with delicacy and finesse. The course of about four to five miles is divided into 18 holes, each having a flat tee where you drive off, a fairway of mown grass, and finishing at a beautifully kept green where the hole is marked by a flag. The object is to get the ball from the tee to the green in as few strokes as possible, and hazards such as ponds, trees, sand pits and gullies are all there to make it as difficult and as interesting as possible.

There are 14 clubs with heads of wood or iron, for different kinds of strokes and surfaces. A beginner can do quite well with two woods and three or four irons in a light canvas bag rented from the club, and you can go on playing for years without much more equipment. One problem may be finding a local course; many of the best courses are private, where you can only play as a member or a member's guest. But there are many public courses open to anyone, especially around cities and towns, and you can telephone ahead to book a time. You will have to pay a green fee.

Women are still not allowed to play on most courses during the weekend until the afternoon, since so many men play on Saturday or Sunday mornings. There are sometimes regulations about young children who are required to have lessons before they go out with you; check ahead of time.

JOINING A CLUB

Private golf clubs are still social as well as sport clubs, and most have strict rules about how to become a member, and who can join. You will probably need to be sponsored by another member, but if you don't know anyone locally, do ask at the club; good players are often welcome.

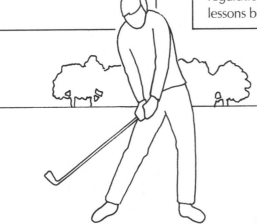

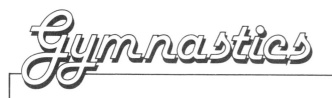

CARTWHEELS ON THE BEAM

Many of us, when we think of gymnastics, think of Olga Korbut and her elegant acrobatics on the balance beam. Like many Olympic sports, it may look too difficult to tackle. But, in fact, gymnastics is so varied that there is sure to be something manageable for even the most abject beginner. It is wonderful exercise for building and toning muscles, and because some of the acrobatics are almost dance-like, it can contribute to more graceful movement and flexibility. It is a perfect exercise routine for training for other sports as well.

Gymnastics is a system of exercising using a variety of apparatus including the vaulting horse, the pommel-horse, alloy rings, parallel bars, asymmetric bars, horizontal or high bars, the balance beam, mats for floor exercises and sometimes a trampoline. You must find a gymnasium that is really equipped. Many YMCA's sponsor gymnastic lessons and schools and health clubs are also useful sources of information.

Gymnastics requires a certain degree of dexterity and strength, even from the start. People over forty should check their health and fitness carefully before they begin, but if they are in good physical shape, there is no reason that they cannot work up a suitable gymnastics regime. Children usually love gymnastics, so this is a sport that might well be taken up by the whole family.

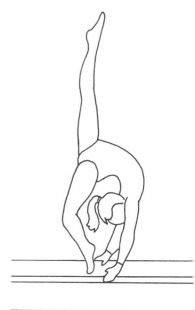

BE CAREFUL

Remember, if you are not properly instructed, injuries or malformation of certain muscles can develop. Don't begin a routine unless an instructor shows you how to use each piece of equipment first.

WHAT YOU NEED, WHERE TO GO, HOW TO LEARN

● A leotard is suitable for women; a snug-fitting exercise suit would work for men

● You should wear gym shoes or ballet slippers, although for some of the exercises, you can be barefoot.

● You don't need guidance all the time you are working out, but you should be instructed correctly in the beginning. Find a class in your neighborhood, at the local school, or youth club, or write to the organization listed in the reference section.

Jumping Rope

SKIPPING TIME

Do you still think jumping rope is for kids? Well, get rid of that picture of pigtailed little girls reciting one-a-penny, two-a-penny as they bounce up and down.

Jumping rope is one of the newest fitness fads, and it looks very much like it's here to stay. There are at least three reasons why jumping is so popular: You can jump anywhere, especially in the privacy of your home. That is important to many people who are out of condition, and a little unhappy about being in the public eye dressed in shorts or track suits. If you have a garden, or a yard, then it's the perfect way to get fresh air, exercise and enjoyment without moving five steps away from the house. So jumping is the answer for young mothers, or anyone housebound who would find it difficult to get away even for half an hour.

It's quick and easy. With no equipment beyond the rope itself, you can start with a few minutes and gradually work up to fifteen minutes or even half an hour. You won't need lessons; the only real problem may be boredom, and then it is back to childhood, counting games, twisting hands, crossing hands and for the family, lots of old-fashioned games with a long rope, two at each end, one in the middle. Jumping is great for cardiovascular efficiency, it gets your whole system toned up and glowing, uses up to 120 calories about every ten minutes, and generally improves the entire body tone. Even more, it's fun!

WORTH NOTING

Children's ropes sometimes have rough handles and too short a length. But, you might find it a little difficult to buy an adult skipping rope, so try a good sports store – they should have suitable ropes made for boxers who skip rope regularly as part of their training.

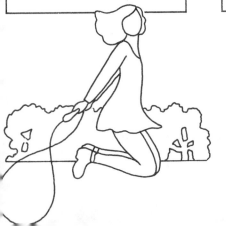

WHAT YOU NEED, WHERE TO GO, HOW TO LEARN

● Wear comfortable, easy-fitting clothes; a track suit is perfect outdoors, a leotard or just a knit shirt and shorts indoors. Tennis shoes are useful.

● The rope itself should be very inexpensive. That's all you need.

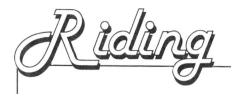

THE WORLD OF HORSES

A horse was once man's car, tractor, and a natural supply of highly organic fertilizer. Horse and rider have been a vital element in the economy and a familiar part of the landscape for thousands of years.

Riding used to be very simple – you jumped on and slid off, perhaps with a cloth to sit on and a halter to hold. Today it is a little more complicated, but it is still the trust and co-operation between horse and rider which is so exciting and satisfying, and so beautiful to watch. Some people are frightened of horses because of their strength and size, but in reality they are very responsive creatures, usually eager for attention and affectionate care. A well-trained horse will turn or trot with only the slightest movement of his rider, so you can begin as a young child, and there's no reason why you shouldn't still be trotting through the countryside at ninety!

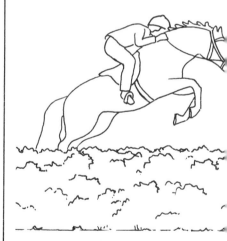

Apart from getting you outside in all weathers – you can find places to ride indoors but it's much less fun – riding is very good for balance, muscular co-ordination, strengthening leg and thigh muscles, and for breathing too. Just riding out is great, exploring trails and bridle paths, but the wide variety of horse sports offers even more fun for the competitive family.

WHAT YOU NEED, WHERE TO GO, HOW TO LEARN

● Heeled and close fitting boots or laced shoes, tight legged trousers, so they won't rub, and a comfortable jacket or sweater will do, but you *must* have a hat. Later you can buy a hacking jacket and riding jodpurs – you'll need them for almost all shows and competitions.

● The one thing that is really vital, of course, is the horse which can be hired by the hour from livery stables. If you want to buy your own animal, be sure you really know what you are taking on, and have a long talk with a local vet about space and conditions. Any horse, even the smallest pony, will need a warm, dry stable, at least a small pasture in which to graze part of the day, and money for all the unexpected expenses – vets' bills, medicines, broken and lost equipment.

GETTING DOWN TO BASICS
Once you can ride, think about
JUNIOR GYMKHANAS
all sorts of racing with obstacles, mostly for the pony club group.
SHOW JUMPING
Basically, a series of jumps in a ring, graded according to size and experience of the horse, and the amount of money the horse has won.
CROSS COUNTRY
Cross country riding over a set course, kept as natural as possible, but with man-made, rustic-looking jumps.

DRESSAGE
Really a test of grace and control. The horse, quiet and beautifully groomed, should always be completely under control.

PONY TREKKING & ENDURANCE
Not really competitive but can be made so by the first home winning the prize.

WORTH NOTING

● Anyone with back trouble, balancing problems or any kind of brittle bone disease must check with their doctor first. But riding seems to be especially good for disabled children and adults, giving a chance of first-class recreation, and encouraging co-ordination as well as increased self-confidence. There are many fine organizations devoted to helping them enjoy every kind of riding.

● So you've bought a hat … well, see you wear it *always*.

● Never underestimate the power of a horse – treat it with respect always, and with caution until you know what you're doing.

● Don't ride on public roads unless taken there by an instructor. Keep to paths that are specially marked for riders, and that often doesn't include footpaths.

● If you must ride at night, make sure you have a luminous strip on both your hat and jacket.

● Except for race horses, a horse isn't ready for regular riding till it's three, for jumping till it's four. Beginners are best on a mount of eight to ten years, steady and quiet.

Saddles

An English saddle is flat and doesn't give a lot of support. The rider must use muscle power to rise and fall – very good for fitness! The Western saddle is designed for range riding, a U shape with a high pommel in front. Most experts feel that English riding, although harder to learn, is absolutely vital if you want to ride well.

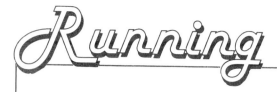

Running

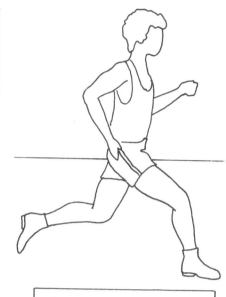

ON THE RUN

Even a few years ago, the only runners you'd normally see on the roads were athletes in training, but today it is practically a national pastime. Doctors, clerks, housewives, young, middle-aged or very senior citizens – they're all out there, finding new enjoyment and physical well-being in simply making a run for it.

If you literally take to the road four or five times a week you'll be giving your heart and lungs all the exercise they need. And at the same time you could be leaving all your troubles behind – running is one of the best ways to get rid of tensions and anxiety.

How fast you run decides whether you're a jogger or not. Do a slow run and you're jogging. If you pit yourself against the clock, aiming for speed, then without question you're definitely a runner! But really it doesn't matter what you call it as long as you get out there and enjoy it.

As far as burning up the calories go, you'll use up almost twice as many sprinting as just jogging (125 calories in ten minutes) but you obviously won't be able to keep it up so long. But you do get more benefit if you sprint now and then.

The wonderful thing about running is that it doesn't require basic sports ability, expensive equipment or even great effort to get organized. You can run anywhere, anytime. And provided you're sensible about it, you can begin at any age.

BEFORE YOU BEGIN ...

● Know when to stop. If you have any warning signs like severe breathlessness, nausea, dizziness, pains in the chest, you've been overdoing it and a medical check-up might be necessary.

● Don't run on main roads, especially if you're going out as a family.

● Never run until at least an hour or so after a meal.

WHAT YOU NEED, WHERE TO GO, HOW TO LEARN

● *Where* you run is up to you. To begin with, it might be nice to find a proper track near your home or office. Parks can provide good running, too. If you have to use the street, make sure you run against the traffic. Even a treadmill at home can be your private track. Dull but useful.

● Some country areas now have special places for runners. It's also worth finding out if your local school has indoor or outdoor jogging facilities. Some may keep open in the evening or at weekends. You don't need lessons as such, but it can help to start out with a more experienced jogger; you'll be able to pick up a host of tips.

START-UP TIME

Always do at least 10 minutes of warming up exercises every time you go for a run. Even something simple like just bending over from your waist, with legs straight, and letting your arms and head relax completely. Leg stretchers are also very helpful.

For the first few minutes of your run, just walk, then go into a slow jog so that your heart and lungs have a chance to adjust to the increasing workload. Go as smoothly as you can – *don't* bounce along – and run flat-footed, not on your toes. Keep your arms bent so that your forearms are nearly parallel to the ground and let them swing backwards and forwards as you go.

Establish your pace, and while that pace may increase in speed, always try to keep your pace steady. Never stop running cold. Always run or walk 'down' or do a few warming down exercises after you have finished your run.

Whatever your age, you shouldn't just suddenly trot off. If you're normally fit with no specific health problems, and under 35, start your first running week by going out three or four times and doing half a mile, alternating 100 paces jogging with 100 paces walking. Next week do the same thing over a distance of one and a half miles. Finally, run a mile comfortably and follow that up a week later by going as fast as you can. But check your pulse rate just after you finish – over 120 beats a minute and you're overdoing it.

● Be sensible. Women running on their own should obviously avoid notorious spots where muggers or rapists have been sighted. It makes sense in city streets to go with others. If you wouldn't walk there on your own then don't run there. And that goes for men, too.

● At night, wear light clothes plus something fluorescent.

● The only item you should buy is a quality pair of running shoes. Tennis, squash or track shoes are fine for beginners, but for a serious runner, shoes are essential. Go to a good sports store.

● Although you might want to buy a regular track suit (they are popular at the moment, so you will have no trouble finding them in stores), it is not essential. Make sure that your pants legs are loose so that they do not chafe. In cooler weather, always wear a sweater and long pants even though you will heat up; improper insulation can cause muscles to tense. A hat, a scarf, and gloves are also needed in really cold weather. Shorts and a tee shirt are all you need to wear in warm weather.

Skateboarding

WHEELS BY THE SET

It has taken the world by storm. An estimated 5000 skateboards are being bought daily in the States and the publicity has been overwhelming. But it's really not new. It almost certainly began in California in the mid sixties. Something like 50 million boards were sold overnight … then nothing, it simply fizzled out. Today, the skateboard has reappeared with a vengeance – and one difference; the early boards could wear out four sets of the old metal wheels daily, but the new plastic ones are much more sturdy.

The fastest speed recorded has been over sixty miles an hour. Not suprisingly, there have been many accidents, and parents have been trying to get safety clothing and rules accepted by their speed-crazed children. It's really a youngster's sport, demanding very good balance and co-ordination. Not for the overweight, but surfers and skiers might try. The calorie cost for ten minutes is moderately high – around 95–100 calories burned away.

A skateboard is a rolling platform to stand on and control by shifting your weight. They can be quite expensive, so they are usually bought by parents, and this is one case where economy doesn't pay, because a crash at high speed can injure a child for life.

Make sure your child wears the protective gear. Falling off the board is almost part of the sport, and heads, arms and knees get broken regularly and often very badly.

WORTH NOTING

● Always wear protective clothing; a helmet, knee and elbow pads, and gloves. Elbow pads are especially important as one of the commonest injuries is a fractured 'funny bone'.

● Check for cracks and wear and tear every time you use your board.

● Not suitable for the children under the age of eight.

● Never go out alone. If you are injured, you should have a companion who can fetch help.

WHAT YOU NEED, WHERE TO GO, HOW TO LEARN

● Sweat suits are ideal, otherwise something comfortable with no trailing bits to get caught under the wheels.

● Flat shoes with rubber soles and reinforced toes, like training or tennis shoes are necessary.

● Choose a recommended skateboard. It will cost more but it will be safer and should last longer too. Get one already assembled. The kits can be unsteady and difficult to tighten sufficiently.

● Go to a supervised park – they are opening all over the place as the craze develops. You may be able to hire all the equipment or find a quiet spot somewhere with a flat surface. Don't go too fast at first and learn to stop and start before anything else.

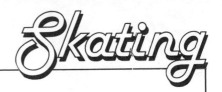

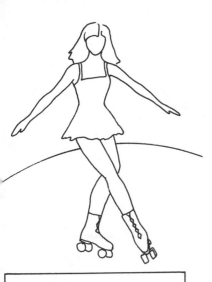

ICE SKATING

Most people skate for fun, but it can also offer all kinds of activities to the enthusiastic skater. Figure skating, alone or in pairs, is an internationally recognized sport. Speed skating is also popular, and it can be enjoyed indoors and outdoors. Ice rinks today cater for all the family; there are often special classes for young children, and sessions for dancers. Most ice rinks have set hours for the public, because the ice must be cleaned and scraped smooth after so many hours use. Telephone ahead to check. Apart from being great recreation, skating is good for co-ordination of movement, balance and control. Ten minutes uses up 115 calories, so it's pretty strenuous.

ROLLER SKATING

Once ice skating had become popular, and before indoor rinks were possible, it seemed a long time to wait between winters. A Dutchman tried putting wheels on instead of blades, and a new sport was invented.

Children love roller skating, and the big advantage has always been being able to walk out the door and get started. There are also races and competitions for the fanatic, especially today when there are far more roller skating rinks than people realize. Check in your area or with the national club.

WORTH NOTING

● See your doctor if you've had ankle trouble or poor balance.

● Never ice-skate on unknown lakes or ponds, unless the ice has been tested first by an expert. Skating on thin ice is no joke.

● Don't let children go ice skating on their own unless it's at a supervised rink.

● Have all skates checked regularly if you own them. Ice skates need sharpening quite often.

WHAT YOU NEED, WHERE TO GO, HOW TO LEARN

● Clothes; opt for comfort rather than glamour. Skate in trousers or a full, short skirt. Tights and an extra pair of socks are useful. Simple roller skates clip on to stout walking shoes with laces and strong soles.

● You can rent skates at any indoor rink, at very reasonable prices. Take along your own socks, though, and a lace hook to help you do them up. When you know this is a sport you want to keep on with, buy your own, and buy the best you can afford. Keep them dry when stored, and protect ice blades with special rubber skids.

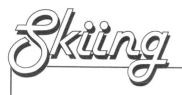

SNOW AND ICE

Despite its trendy image, skiing has a long history. A 4,000-year-old rock carving in Norway shows a man holding a stick, and standing on very long skis. Of course, skiing was an essential form of transportation then in any country where snow was on the ground most of the year. And when snowfalls block our roads and stop cars and buses, skiing can still be the easiest and quickest way to get around.

Most skiers are interested more in enjoyment, and it is now one of the most popular leisure sports throughout the world. Ski resorts have been built wherever there is a chance of snow.

There are two basic kinds of skiing – Alpine, or downhill, and Nordic, or cross-country. It can be highly competitive, and the Olympic races are really exciting to watch. But one of the best points is that anyone can join in from the middle aged to the toddler. Children can learn to ski as soon as they can walk, and grandparents can slip comfortably and easily through a crowd of teen-aged beginners just learning clumsily how to turn. Most good resorts encourage every age group, and provide slopes for all levels of expertise; and the sociability and night life after dark make it enjoyable for single people too. Warm sun, crisp snow, clean air – the perfect sport.

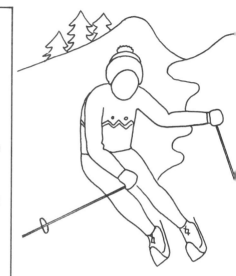

GETTING STARTED

If you don't live near a suitable resort or ski slope, it might be simpler to try cross-country skiing first as long as the snowfall is reasonably deep.

If you are in the country, carry a compass and never go out alone; the snow makes ordinary landmarks disappear, and when the landscape is all white, it's all too easy to get lost.

WHAT YOU NEED, WHERE TO GO, HOW TO LEARN

Clothes must be warm, and preferably layered; a light sweater, a heavier sweater, a waterproof ski jacket, waterproof pants, warm socks, gloves, and goggles, and cap. Tights underneath the pants are an extra protection on cold days, for men as well as women.

• Cross-country skiers often wear shorter trousers with long heavy knee socks that leave the leg free.

• Always rent your skis, boots and poles when you begin; they are expensive to buy and clumsy to carry on the trip. Most resorts will give you the basic charge for ski hire, the pass for the ski lifts and the lessons. Private lessons will be more, and you will probably have to reserve an instructor in advance.

BOOTS

Boots are an important part of your equipment. Heavy downhill boots hold the foot firmly and flat on the ski. Clips are easier than old-fashioned laces, and the bindings which hold the shoe must be checked often to be sure they will fall off if you twist your foot too much; otherwise you can break an ankle.

Cross-country boots are much lighter, they tie like a shoe, and slip into toe bindings which leave the heel free.

Both boots can be hired at the resort, but when you become a regular skier, they are the first piece of equipment to buy. Badly fitting boots can be agony.

ALPINE OR DOWNHILL SKIING

This is the most challenging kind of skiing, and the most well-known. You'll begin on low nursery slopes, learning to manipulate the long skis, using your poles to balance yourself rather than push you along, and managing to stay upright for most of the time. Short skis are a new idea for real beginners, as they are much easier to handle. Less calories are burnt up than cross country, about 90 for ten minutes skiing.

As you improve, you'll move up to steeper slopes, but always keep to the routes marked for your level of skill. If you stray off prepared runs, you may be badly hurt, so pay attention to the signs.
Expert skiers can choose almost any slope, but even then don't overestimate your skill; cold, sleet and an unexpected avalanche can be dangerous enemies.

CROSS COUNTRY OR NORDIC SKIING

Entirely different, cross country skiing has very different techniques and benefits. It's a high-energy sport, burning up 125 calories in ten minutes. You move across relatively flat ground, propelling yourself with poles and long, almost skating, glides. It's particularly good for building strong leg muscles, and although it may not be as exciting as downhill, you can go cross-country anywhere — fields, meadows, in a forest, or on snow-covered city streets.

● Don't try to learn alone; it helps enormously to be with a group of similar skill – or lack of it – and it will keep you from overdoing it. That is when accidents happen.

● Do some pre-ski exercises before you go to limber up unused muscles. It will pay dividends in extra days of enjoyment.

● Write to the national organization for recommended resorts and package trips, which are very popular with all skiers, and the best value.

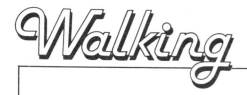

Walking

ON YOUR FEET

It may seem odd to include walking as a 'sport', but in fact, walking is one of the easiest and best ways to keep yourself trim and healthy. Moreover, more than any other sport, walking has the least restriction. Anyone can walk – the young, the old, busy or lazy, those in the best of health or many of those recuperating from illness. You can walk any time of year – an easy stroll on a summer evening is a delight, a brisk walk on a winter morning is stimulating. Finally, you can walk any place. If you live in the city, a quick walk can ease tensions. (In addition, it may often be easier to walk than to fight traffic.) If you live in a suburban area or in the country, walking is a wonderful way to enjoy the sights and smells of nature.

With regard to walking as exercise, it is best to consider it a habit to be cultivated. In other words, get in the habit of walking whenever and wherever you can. Instead of hopping into your car to get a bottle of milk, walk to the corner, instead of riding to the station, walk!

Unlike more vigorous sports such as skiing or jogging, you can't plan on losing weight simply by walking, but you will be surprised at how, over a period of months, those few extra calories you burn up each day will result in slow weight loss. In addition, your leg muscles will be firmer and the increased blood circulation will give your skin a healthy glow and all your organs added vitality.

Walking While Travelling

Another way both to get your required exercise and to learn about places you visit is to walk as much as possible whenever you travel. Many cities include walking tours as a large part of their local tourist business. The travel office of nearly every city in the world will provide city maps and suggested walks to city visitors. Most of the walks will, of course, include famous sights, and they can lead to exciting discoveries.

WHAT YOU NEED, WHERE TO GO, HOW TO LEARN

• Sturdy, comfortable, shoes are the only requirement. Walking in high heels or tight shoes is not only uncomfortable it can be damaging to your feet and back

• Keep an open mind while you are walking. If you are observing sights around you, wherever you may be, stay alert. If you are walking merely to relax, relax your mind as well as your body.

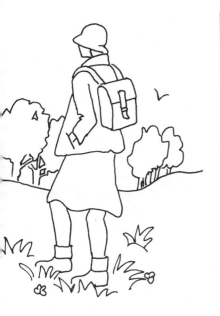

Walking can often be a fine activity for mental health. Many people find that they do their best thinking while taking a walk. Walking can require no concentration at all, but the mild exercise combined with a subtle change of scenery can free the mind to solve a problem. On the other hand, while walking, you can concentrate on flowers, or sunshine, or shop windows, and give your mind something fresh to think about.

Walking as Sport
In some senses, walking can be considered a sport, but because it is not physically demanding, it should be used in concert with other hobbies. Bird watching and other forms of nature studies, for example, are usually done on foot. If you enjoy photography, an infinite number of wonderful potential pictures can be found even on the shortest walk.

Walking can – and often does – become the primary form of exercise for older people, (and sometimes for those who are not so old). If this is the case, walking should, again, become a disciplined habit. A walk of specified distance and for a specific amount of time should be taken at least once a day. For example, an evening walk around the block or for one mile down a road should become a part of a daily routine. An excellent time to walk is after a meal; any meal will do – breakfast, lunch, or dinner. Keep a sense of timing; in other words, begin with half an hour for a two-mile walk. Don't rush, but don't dawdle either. Two walks per day, of course, are even better than one.

FOR ALL OF US

Walking, over the long term and if you train yourself to walk often and regularly, is fine exercise. It is not demanding physically, you can do it any time and any place, and you will keep your body and mind running smoothly.

Water Sports

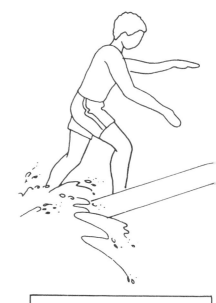

SURFING

It's one of those things that *looks* easy – lying or standing on a board in the sea and then riding into the shore on the crest of a wave. But it's not easy to master – though once you have, surfing can be a really fantastic sport. Basically, it's from Hawaii which is enough to recommend it for lots of people and for fairly obvious reasons is a summer sport only.

It's pretty good all-round exercise as far as developing muscles, flexibility and relieving tensions are concerned but for co-ordination of movement it's first class. You won't be burning up those calories though – you'll be lucky to lose 70 in ten minutes.

Surfing can be quite dangerous. Remember that what comes in must go out. In other words, every wave that sweeps to shore has to flow out again, and on some beaches these ebbing waters can be very strong. Look out for strong waters before you begin. Should you ever get caught and find yourself being drawn back to sea, try to keep calm, check your breathing and then start swimming parallel to the shore until you're out of the ebb tide area. Then you'll find it easier to swim in the right direction.

Surf on recommended beaches only. You must be a strong swimmer. Some experts recommend that you should be able to swim strongly for at least 150 yards in the sea, as well as being strong enough to control a surfboard while paddling out through severe breaking waves.

WORTH NOTING

● Never go surfing alone.

● Never let your surfboard float free. It could be very dangerous if it hits you or another surfer.

● Keep your board in good repair.

● Not suitable for young children or for anyone past middle age.

WHAT YOU NEED, WHERE TO GO, HOW TO LEARN

● Not much equipment is required: a swimsuit and a surfboard. You can often hire the surfboard at the beach.

● You obviously need a sea shore with strong waves.

● Write to the national organization for beaches with instructors or equipment.

186

LOOK OUT FOR …

• It's for swimmers only, and always wear a life jacket until you really know what you are doing.

• Learn the right hand signals and rehearse them with the boat's helmsman and any passengers *before* going out on the skis.

• Always check *all* the equipment thoroughly for any faults before going out.

• Always watch the water ahead of you.

• Remember to let go of the tow handle right away if you fall over. Don't forget to let the helmsman know you're OK by holding up your hand.

• The wake from other boats can be dangerous, so watch out for motorboats (and swimmers!) too close for comfort.

WATER SKIING

Although it looks very daring, water skiing is regarded as the perfect family sport because almost anyone, even a child, can pick up enough skill to enjoy themselves. In its present form it is fairly new, although its origins lie in surfboarding, which has been around for generations. With the invention of the motor boat in 1885, the sport took another leap forward when it became aqua-planing – the board was towed with the rider standing. Finally, the board was divided into two to become skis and the sport, as we know it, was born.

The training period is short, the sport is easily learned and you start enjoying yourself almost right from the start. It doesn't use up a great deal of energy either – you'd use up only 65 calories in ten minutes, just five more than a walk. But it is good for co-ordination of movement and will also help to develop certain muscles. Some handicapped people can enjoy it too – even the blind, as long as the boat towing the skier is careful to avoid obstacles.

A club should supply the special skis (which need expert fitting) plus boat and 75 foot tow lines, and a tow with two types of handles – single or double. As a beginner you would use a double.

WHAT YOU NEED, WHERE TO GO, HOW TO LEARN

• You'll need an ordinary swimsuit in warm weather but a rubber suit is more practical in cool climates.

• You will need lessons from a qualified teacher. Join a club, or ask for a trial lesson. Most clubs observe local regulations and have a licence.

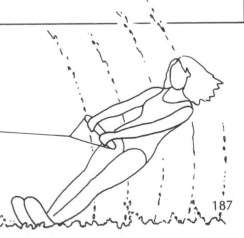

SWIMMING AND DIVING

The ancient Egyptians loved it and it was part of the basic training for the Roman armies. So swimming certainly isn't new, and it has stayed one of the most popular family sports, with the pleasure of remembering warm summer days at the beach all through the cold winter.

Today, with quite a few indoor pools available at schools and leisure areas, its much more of a year-round possibility. Just in case you don't know, swimming is basically a way of propelling yourself through water. Apart from the obvious life-saving advantages, it's also wonderful exercise for lungs, muscles and heart – you can't swim properly without breathing hard and deeply. And you'll burn up around 100 calories for every ten minutes' activity.

Swimming can improve the figure, too – building up the lean person and breaking down the fatty tissues in the not-so-lean. In fact it's about the only sport where a really over-weight person won't be handicapped, because the water literally takes the strain and holds up your body.

Swimming styles can be adapted to suit the needs of the disabled. For this you must have skilled help and guidance. There are all sorts of special aids available nowadays which can help even the most severely handicapped find some enjoyment. Swimming is also excellent for strengthening weak spines and it's one of the few sports recommended for people with weak hearts – with medical permission only, of course.

SWIMMING – LOOK OUT FOR ...

● Never swim alone, or without someone nearby. It only takes a few minutes to drown.

● Allow at least two hours after a meal or you could get chronic stomach cramps. Just as important, don't go in when you're really hungry or very tired.

● Never go swimming when the tide is going out or there's any kind of warning flag flying. Swim along the coastline, never out to sea.

● If you suffer from any kind of ear trouble, consult your doctor.

● Know the right time to come out! It should be when you feel your best, not when you're beginning to get chilled.

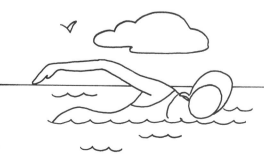

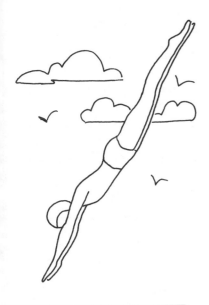

GETTING DOWN TO BASICS

Just splashing about doesn't count as far as real exercise is concerned, although it's a marvellous way to let children enjoy being in the water. Paddling pools are always popular, but remember that a child can drown in only a few inches of water – even more reason for seeing that everyone in the family knows how to float and swim. For older people, the fitness benefits are large; every single part of the body gets a first-class workout.

DIVING

Once you can swim you might want to learn how to dive – a far more attractive and interesting way of getting into the water than creeping down the pool steps. It's even better for your lungs, and helps produce steady nerves and good co-ordination at the same time, though as weight reducing exercise, it's only half as productive as swimming – just 50 calories in ten minutes. But there's a great deal of difference between what you could expect to do at the local pool and competition level diving. Top divers use high platforms or springboards over extremely deep diving pools, and make a series of somersaults and twists before reaching the water. Obviously something you can't just pick up over night … with all diving you need proper instruction and the right facilities.

DIVING – LOOK OUT FOR …

● Never attempt even the simplest dive in a crowded pool, or into the sea.

● Always have proper instruction – a belly flop can be very painful.

● Always check the depth of the diving area – you need at least seven feet of water for simple dives from the edge of the pool.

WHAT YOU NEED, WHERE TO GO, HOW TO LEARN

● In most public areas, you'll all need swimsuits, but the classic tank suits or shorts are the most efficient and usually the cheapest. Some 'swimsuits' are so fashionably cut they are only for show. Keep them for sunbathing. Swimwear should be comfortable, not needing a lot of attention … like bikini straps that keep falling down. You may have to wear a cap at some pools and it will also protect your hair from the pool's strong chemicals.

● A small local pool is the safest bet for beginners. The sea is fine if you follow basic safety regulations.

Doubling Up

DOUBLING UP

So far, we've covered a good many sports you can do on your own. But if you don't enjoy getting out by yourself, or if your fitness campaign is a joint family effort, then it is a good idea to look at the pair sports which need two or more players.

When both sports partners are beginners, or experts, then there will be no problem. If the difference in skill isn't too much, then use a handicap system to let the duffer have a bit of a chance. In any case, it usually improves your game to play with someone better than yourself. However, if there is a very wide variation in skill, then you'll have to pick your sport more carefully. Look for a game where luck and energy can help.

Don't forget ballroom dancing; it's not quite a sport but in terms of exercise and fitness it's top value for any couple, plus a good way to put a little sparkle in your social life.

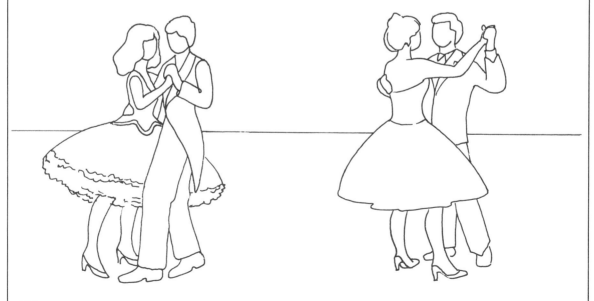

Badminton

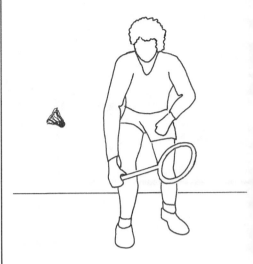

SHUTTLECOCKS AND RACKETS

Badminton is played on a marked court, 44' × 20'. The net is 5' high, and the smallish flexible rackets are very lightweight, about 3–5 ounces depending on size. The shuttlecock was made traditionally with sixteen 2" goose feathers firmly embedded in a cork ball - today it's usually plastic.

Badminton can be played as singles or doubles. The shuttlecock is hit across the net, aimed at the floor on the other side and it must be returned before it touches the floor. Only the serving side can score, getting one point on winning the rally. If the server loses, then the opposite side serves. The first to make 15 points (11 in women's tournaments) wins the game.

In a leisurely family game you can start to enjoy yourself very quickly. The racket is so light that young and old can join in. It can be played indoors all the year round, although on a quiet summer's day it is lovely to have an outside match, and it's the ideal family game for the garden, burning up 85 calories in ten minutes play for the over weight.

Badminton scores pretty well for all-round exercise and gets top marks for physical recreation. There is a wide range of strokes – and with some of the overhead smashes it is possible to get the shuttlecock on its way at an estimated speed of 90 mph. It gives you great co-ordination of movement.

WORTH NOTING

● The equipment is so light that new players forget that badminton can be very strenuous, so take it easy at the beginning.

● Wrist control is essential. If you have any weakness, check with your doctor first.

WHAT YOU NEED, WHERE TO GO, HOW TO LEARN

● Normal tennis clothes – shorts or a skirt, and shirt, socks and shoes. For family games on the lawn, play in anything comfortable. Clubs are more likely to ask you to wear white, so check before you join.

● Although badminton rackets are cheaper than tennis rackets, they can be expensive especially with a press to keep the frame straight. Steel rackets are more to buy but do not need a press.

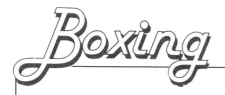

Boxing

IN THE RING

Boxing has a reputation for brutality, but considering that men used to box with no gloves on and the audience often joined in the fight, the 'Golden Gloves' have come a long way. Today despite the bloody image, boxing comes only tenth in the sports league of injuries.

Boys' clubs have always encouraged boxing for self-discipline and as an acceptable way of working off aggressive feelings. Amateur bouts are carefully supervised, with skill and general alertness getting top points.

The referee sees that the rules are observed, and 'seconds' look after the fighters at the end of each round – sponge them down and repair any cuts, etc. Boxers are also matched by weight, so a skinny 5'3" boy won't be expected to tackle a heavy-framed 6' opponent.

It is a young person's game and amateurs should really hang up their gloves by the time they are thirty. But for fitness fanatics a few minutes boxing is worth hours of another sport – punching a bag for just ten minutes can use up 225 calories! And you can go on sparring (with extra-thick gloves, practising rather than really punching) for half an hour at a time, for many years.

WARNING

● No one with a squint, or tendencies to epilepsy, however mild, should box. If there's a history of heart disease in your family, have a check-up. Regular sight tests are recommended for everyone.

WHAT YOU NEED, WHERE TO GO, HOW TO LEARN

● Gloves are essential, weighing at least twelve ounces for beginners, to soften and spread the blows. Special bandages will tape up hands, and a gumshield protects the teeth. Men need an athletic supporter, and women a padded undershirt for their breasts.

● Professional support shoes are recommended, but shorts and a tee shirt are fine. Keep a sweatshirt handy for after the bout.

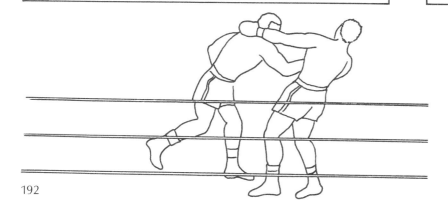

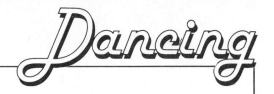

LET'S DANCE

When the music starts to play, most of us would like to get up and dance. Dancing seems to be a natural human activity, and since it has been recorded in every culture of the world since the beginning of history, it must have an important place in human development and culture.

Today it has lost most of its formal ritual, but dancing has remained an enormous pleasure for untold millions. Every decade, every generation, has had its special dance music and dance steps. Traditional ballroom dancing from the days of Fred Astaire is still popular, and there are dance halls in many towns and cities which are open to everyone. Discotheques are popular with the younger generation, and they are the best places to learn the latest routines and the newest and most exciting steps.

Then there are dozens of kinds of country and folk dancing clubs which are usually only too happy to have new members – enthusiasm and good spirits are all you need.

Dancing is for anyone, at any age. You can make it as strenuous or as quietly elegant as you like, depending on your tastes and the company; you may not burn up huge amounts of calories, but if you really enjoy yourself, take a few lessons if you need them, and dance regularly, then you can develop a good sense of coordination, balance, and smooth movement.

SHOWING OFF

In addition to informal parties, there are displays and exhibitions of many dance teams – country dances, Highland reels, South American congas – everything you can think of. Ask at the dance school or dance hall for information. You will probably have to provide your own costume and expenses when you travel, but it's an energetic way to meet new friends.

WHAT YOU NEED, WHERE TO GO, HOW TO LEARN

• At classes, wear anything comfortable which allows easy movement, and well-fitting shoes. For an evening out, most dance halls encourage men to wear a jacket and tie, but at discotheques everything from jeans to slinky satin will be fine.

• Most towns and cities have dancing schools; look in the telephone directory. Lessons aren't strictly necessary, but it's a good way to get started.

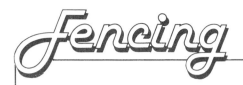

Fencing

FOILS AND SABRES

It used to be a question of gentlemanly behavior, the aristocratic way to settle an argument. If insulted or offended you drew your sword and challenged your opponent. When gentlemen switched to pistols for such matters, foils became less important as weapons, and fencing itself developed into the most graceful of all fighting sports. Foils are the most popular, with a flexible blade and flat guard. Epées have a bowl-shaped guard and a rigid blade. Today it is really an art, requiring good balance and posture – and it's very good for straightening out those round shoulders.
It may not burn away all that many calories – only 75 in ten minutes play – but it encourages co-ordination and graceful movement, and it is excellent as a back-up for other sports like tennis which also need quick, well-balanced movements on the court.
Modern fencing duels take place on almost any flat surface, which is marked in a long rectangle as the duelling area. It's not like being Errol Flynn – you must keep within the specified boundaries, you cannot throw your foil from hand to hand, and swinging from chandeliers is definitely frowned on.
But it is an exciting sport, beautiful to watch, suitable for everyone in the family, and really first class as all-round exercise. Since endurance is not important compared to skill and suppleness, older players can keep on for a very long time.

WORTH NOTING

Always handle the foils with care, although there are buttons on the end. Wear gloves or hold them by the hilt. There are certain target areas on the body for every kind of swordplay – a touch is enough to score the point. Not for people with distorted vision, but disabled players have developed new wheelchair techniques, and they have teams for special Olympic competitions.

WHAT YOU NEED, WHERE TO GO, HOW TO LEARN

● Masks, padded jackets and trousers, and gloves are all a must. Hire them to begin with when you hire your foil.

● Men and women both have special protective undergarments.

● Classes are often taught at YMCA's or athletic clubs. You must have an instructor. You might try the local drama school – some have coaches for classical productions. Get in touch with the national organization for more information.

UNARMED COMBAT

'The martial arts' including Judo, Karate, and Tai Chi are becoming increasingly popular as more and more people want to be able to copy Kung Fu movie stars, and protect themselves at the same time. In the East, all the martial arts are for self-discipline of the mind, and only incidentally about self defence. However, they are excellent all-round physical training … and you probably won't be aware of the good it is doing simply because they require a lot of concentration. You're likely to burn up almost as many calories as you would swimming, about 90 for every ten minutes of activity. You can't keep going for hours, though, and it isn't intended to build up muscles.

Basically, the martial arts are forms of defence used to control and divert an attacker's energy. Most of us have visions of people in pyjamas wrestling on a mat, but there's a lot more to it than that and there are set formalities involved which mean you shouldn't get hurt. In any case, you learn how to fall properly when thrown.

All the family can learn, although children normally don't start until about eight. Very aggressive teenagers can become hooked, so encourage it eagerly – all the martial arts are socially accepted and enjoyable ways of putting restless physical energy to good use.

An important plus for girls and women: a basic knowledge of judo or karate is good protection against muggers or unwanted attention.

BEFORE YOU BEGIN

• Always go to an authorized instructor. One of the organisations at the back of the book will put you in touch. It can be dangerous to learn from an amateur.

• Anyone with back trouble must take precautions. Check with your doctor.

• Ask for a trial lesson – then you will know if it is really for you.

WHAT YOU NEED, WHERE TO GO, HOW TO LEARN

• A special kind of loose trousers and jacket are worn. Buy them through the club you join or look out for a second-hand pair.

• Lessons are a must, it is not something you can learn from a book. Best bet is to join a club or night school class.

RACKETS

Squash is a game for the fit only, so if you want to play, and you are out of condition, spend at least three weeks limbering up with an assortment of exercises. Once you are fit, though, you will stay that way if you keep playing; squash packs a good deal of energy into every second, you won't have to devote hours and hours to your quest for fitness. You'll burn up over 100 calories in just ten minutes play.

There is no net. Both players face the high front wall, and serve hard so that the ball careens off the sides or the floor, making it impossible for the other player to hit it back.

The rackets are lighter and smaller than tennis rackets; the ball travels very fast, and is difficult to see. Remember you can practice alone. You can go along to a squash court and just keep hitting the ball until you get your strokes right.

Rules vary, depending on whether you are playing British or American squash. For instance, in the British game only the person serving can score, and a winning shot by his opponent means that he can then take over serving. In America, every point counts for the player who hits the winning ball. Size of court varies too. The British court is wider than the American one but it is still basically the same. Another important difference is that the British squash ball weighs less than the American one and the rackets are lighter, too.

WORTH NOTING

● It is certainly a young person's game, unless you have been playing for years.

● Make sure you are really in good condition before you start playing. It is one of the most dangerous sports for the unfit. Doctors say too many out-of-condition men die on the squash courts from heart attacks.

WHAT YOU NEED, WHERE TO GO, HOW TO LEARN

● As far as clothes are concerned, it doesn't really matter what you wear as long as it's white. Tennis clothes – white shorts, skirt, socks and shoes – are most suitable. You must never wear shoes with black soles as they could mark the court.

● Don't buy equipment until you have had several games; squash rackets are certainly not cheap. You should be able to hire rackets and balls, which have to be a special weight. If you do decide to buy, get expert guidance.

Remember you can practice alone. You can go along to a squash court and just keep hitting the ball until you get your strokes right.

Squash is by far the most tiring of all racket sports. It requires a combination of speed, endurance and incredible concentration. You can't take your eyes off the ball for a second. If you do, you will be amazed by how quickly the points mount up against you! Many fans say it is so relaxing because it makes demands not just physically, but mentally, too. It is not really surprising that squash games are usually limited to half hour sessions!

HANDS ONLY

Handball provides the same quality of exercise as squash. But the basic difference is that it lacks the speed and you don't use a racket. As its name implies, you use your hand.

Again, the game is played in a walled court, generally with two players, but it is possible to play doubles. The principle of the game is the same as squash: you hit the ball t to make it bounce in such a way that your opponent won't be able to send it back. It is still very good exercise, damanding a high degree of skill of movement and, interestingly, although it isn't so constantly energetic as squash you are likely to burn up more calories in ten minutes' handball – about 125.

• Don't play just after a meal – allow a good two to three hours.

• Know when to stop; there is a good reason why courts are hired for short periods.

• Do warming up exercises before you begin to stretch and loosen your body. Otherwise you are likely to get torn muscles.

Although you don't need a press, you'll need a rubberized waterproof cover.

• Get someone who knows the game to go through the basic strokes with you. Then just keep on hitting that ball. Try to find someone a little bit better than you are to play with regularly.

• Games are played in clubs and your best bet is to contact one of the organizations at the back of the book if you don't know of any facilities locally or ask at your nearest gym. Some schools have courts that can be used at night or at weekends.

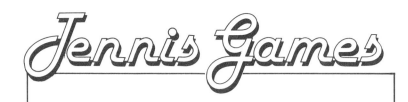

LAWN TENNIS

Even though he had a kingdom and six wives, Henry the Eighth found time to build a tennis court, still in use at Hampton Court. That was the traditional real tennis. Lawn tennis as we know it has only been around since the end of the last century. Grass rectangular courts became a necessary part of any well-appointed country mansion, and white flannel trousers for men and white dresses for women appeared in almost every Noel Coward comedy of the 1930s.

Today it's a very different scene; tennis championships are one of the biggest spectator sports, leading players have fan clubs like movie stars, and the easily-damaged grass surface is often replaced by clay or asphalt, indoors or out, so that avid players can continue their game no matter what the weather or the time of year.

Public courts in many areas have helped to get rid of the snobbish image, and most are available to anyone for hire by the hour. Schools often have tennis teams so that youngsters of all ages are encouraged to learn, and tennis schools and clubs have practice facilities for learners and experts alike.

Watching the great tennis stars in action is a good way of finding out why this exciting, fast-moving game has won over so many new fans, but basically that will exercise your neck, not the rest of you. So get out on the court and play.

WORTH NOTING

If you haven't played for a while, or you are just beginning, don't get into a hard- and-fast singles match right away. Get into shape with home exercises for a few weeks, and start off with doubles, which are easier on all the players. Wrist control is important – if you've had trouble in the past, check with your doctor, and wear an elastic wrist support as extra protection. Never play after a large meal.

WHAT YOU NEED, WHERE TO GO, HOW TO LEARN

● Even today players usually wear white, a knit shirt and shorts or a skirt. You must have good tennis shoes. Buy the best you can afford, because they are useful for almost every kind of sport.
● Rackets and balls are usually owned by the players, but most clubs and gyms do have a few spare ones for real beginners. When you buy your own, get professional advice – rackets can be cheap and cheerful, or *very very* expensive. Youngsters can buy inexpensive junior rackets which are smaller and easier to handle.

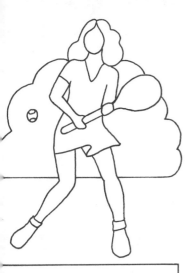

PLATFORM TENNIS

A new craze, Platform Tennis uses a small net-enclosed court on a wooden platform, paddles instead of rackets, and a bright ball bounced off the walls as well as the court. Because it is not as strenuous as ordinary tennis, players can vary widely in age and skill without spoiling the game.

GETTING STARTED

Tennis is one of the most demanding sports, and for reasonably good players, it is strenuous and athletic, burning up 100 calories for every ten minutes of play.
Running around the court, stretching for the ball, spinning around to take a backhand shot or sprinting forward to smash over the net - every muscle in your body will get a good workout.
It is played with two opponents as singles, or with four, as doubles. The court is marked into quarters, with a 3-foot net across the middle. All games start with a diagonal serve across the net, and the basic principle is simply to hit the ball with your racket back and forth, keeping all the bounces within the lines.

The rules are easy to pick up as you play, but it is important to get instruction at the beginning. That will set you off on the right track, and teach you how to hold the racket properly, how to serve, and so on. You can practise on your own against a blank wall.

Especially in doubles, a stronger player can protect a weaker one, so make sure the two best players are on opposite sides of the net. Sometimes a very powerful server can dominate the whole game, so it is important to remember that for sport and exercise winning matches is not the best goal — keep the ball in play as long as you can, volleying back and forth so that everybody has a chance to try out new shots.

- If you really get interested and you have a flat piece of lawn, buy a regulation net and posts to put up at home. Even if space is limited, you can have a lot of fun batting the ball back and forth.

- There are a surprising number of courts around, in city parks as well as private clubs. Go along and find out about the regulations if you want to join a club, and make sure they have facilities for beginners. Most public courts can be hired by the hour, and many have instructors, too, to get you started.

TABLE TOPS

You might wonder why a game remembered from rainy childhood afternoons should be included in a sports book. But you were playing Ping Pong, a very simplified table tennis. At competition level table tennis is fantastically fast, with all sorts of championships and tournaments being held all over the world.

It's an all-year-round indoor sport either with two players as a singles game or four for doubles. The tiny ball is hit with a small paddle over a net that divides a 9-foot long table, in the hope your opponent won't be able to get it back to you. You win one point each time the ball is missed, or isn't returned onto the table on your side of the net.

In fact, it's a bit like a miniature game of lawn tennis. But one big difference is that the ball must always be allowed to bounce before you can hit it. A game is won by the first player to have 21 points, unless both of them get to 20. Then the first to get two points ahead wins. You change over the service every five points, and you change ends of the table after each game. A match consists of either one game, the best of three or the best of five games.

Of course, because it can be easily learned its a good family sport, and be prepared for your kids to beat you once they get the knack of moving quickly. Even at this level, a few games can be first class recreation, and perfect for encouraging hand and eye co-ordination.

MAKING SPACE

The most important requirement is space. Although the table isn't too big, you need quite a lot of clear space at either end in order to play. That little ball goes flying high and wide, and reaching across chairs or around pieces of furniture can cause nasty accidents.

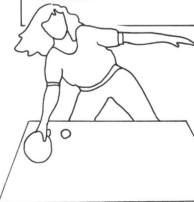

WHAT YOU NEED, WHERE TO GO, HOW TO LEARN

• The one thing not worn is white; dark shirt and shorts are usual with tennis shoes, or anything that's comfortable.

• The table is dark green, nine feet by five, quartered in white. But there are tops you can buy to fit over a dining table, or make a slightly smaller version eight by four fixed to a base. Clubs and gyms often have three or four tables for their members.

• Most people pick up enough skill to play without lessons, and enjoy a game with the family.

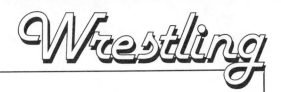

Wrestling

WORTH NOTING

It is basically a young people's sport, not the thing to take up in middle age. But you can probably get away with it until fifty if you started young.

WHAT YOU NEED, WHERE TO GO, HOW TO LEARN

- Most wrestlers wear a tight-fitting one-piece outfit – a bit like an old-fashioned swimsuit – plus athletic supporter. Shoes mustn't have nailed soles, heels, rings or buckles. At home bare feet are fine.

- Some floor covering is used, a large mat or a springy carpet will do.

- You must be taught: it's not something you can pick up from books.

HAND TO HAND

If you lived in a jungle with wild beasts lurking behind every tree, chances are you would learn wrestling with no trouble! Most of us think of wrestling as a grown-up version of puppy fights. Basically, it is the art of keeping an opponent pinned to the ground using only your bare hands. But, of course, it's not quite as simple as that – for there are so many different styles of the sport, all with their own particular rules.

In the Orient, wrestlers have developed an unique and imposing presence, often huge men who go through religiously-controlled training, and a performance is as much a ritual as a spectacular sport.

There are two basic forms of wrestling in the West, Greco-Roman and free form. Greco-Roman contestants must not use thier legs to help them throw thier opponent. In all wrestling, both shoulders on the mat for a count of three signifies a fall.

Whichever style takes your fancy, one thing is for sure – you couldn't find a better sport for developing your muscle power. And it's also pretty good exercise all round, improving stamina, flexibility, co-ordination of movement. It's not too much of a calorie-burner - only 90 calories in ten minutes. It is normally thought of as a man's sport but there is no reason why women shouldn't participate.

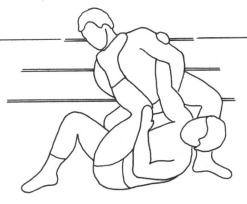

Teaming Up

GROUP SPORTS

There's nothing quite like being part of a team — that sense of belonging, of all pulling together. Of course, finding a team isn't as easy as finding just one friend for tennis.

Look at the noticeboard at your office; many companies have sports clubs, and encourage their staff to get together. If you're at home with young children, then see if your school or church group has some kind of team club. Walk into the local gym or YMCA and see what they have to offer.

You might consider starting your own team. Older children often have friends of their own and it might be quite a lot of fun to make up a group with parents and children playing together, even in competition. But don't be surprised if the children win!

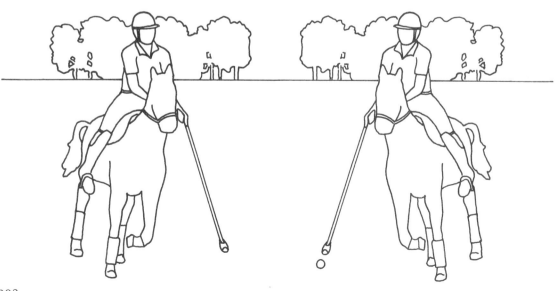

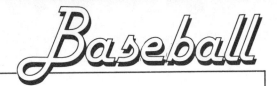

Baseball

BATTING TIME

Despite its all-American image, baseball is a popular summer sport in Europe, particularly in Holland and Italy, and in Middle and South America as well. It is likely that it was based on the game of 'rounders' still played by girls in the majority of English schools.

Baseball is played on a field marked out in a diamond; one point is the batter's home base, and the pitcher is inside the diamond.

There are nine players on each team and the teams play alternatively. One team lines up to bat, while the other is on the field with a pitcher, a catcher, three basemen on each of the corners of the diamond and four fielders. The pitcher in the middle throws the ball towards the batter who has three chances to hit the ball before he is 'out.' If he hits the ball, he must run around the diamond, touching all three bases and returning to home plate. If he makes it all the way around before the ball (or he) is caught, he is said to have hit a 'home run.' If not, he stays on one of the bases, and waits for the next batter to give him a chance to run.

The running in baseball is good exercise, but not terribly strenuous. (You burn up on an average of 50 calories for 10 minutes of play.) It's a great game, though, for all ages.

BEFORE YOU BEGIN

• Swinging the bat around in the air is a good warm-up, but make sure no one is near enough to get hurt.

• Teams may have uniforms, but for casual playing, comfortable slacks and sweat shirts are fine.

• Don't play in icy conditions.

WHAT YOU NEED, WHERE TO GO, HOW TO LEARN

• Baseball bats come in different weights to suit size and skill; most clubs have enough bats and balls to choose from.

• Gloves vary in size and according to use – a catcher's mitt is different from a fielder's glove. Borrow one until you find out what you'll play on the team.

• Baseball shoes have cleats, but tennis shoes are fine.

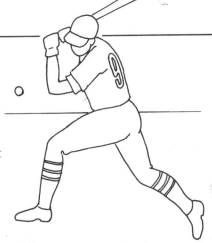

Basketball

BASKETBALL

A social-minded Victorian clergyman tried to invent a game that could be played indoors, outdoors, and all year round to keep young children and teenagers off the streets. His effort was certainly worthwhile, and there are very few schools which don't have a basketball net somewhere.

It's still an exciting team game, played with five team members on each side, on a hard-surfaced court. Tall poles at each end carry a backboard with a ring and net; each team tries to get the large, softish ball through the other team's net, at the same time defending their net from the other team. Players move around a lot, bouncing the ball – (holding is not allowed) and it certainly pays to be tall as the net is 10 feet above the ground – professional basketball players are almost always well over six feet. Scoring is so many points for each time the ball is netted, and games are won by points scored, or sometimes by the clock and the highest score at that time wins.

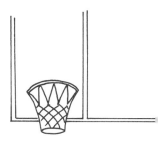

Basketball is pretty strenuous, but it pays off in a reasonably high 110 calories burned in ten minutes. It makes sense as a recreation exercise, too, encouraging good coordination, muscle flexibility and stamina.

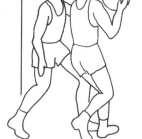

WHAT YOU NEED, WHERE TO GO, HOW TO LEARN

● There are teams and clubs all over for both sports – and many firms have their own teams. Most Gyms and Schools have courts and balls, so you shouldn't have to buy equipment as such.

● Rubber-soled shoes, shorts and a T-shirt are usual and you may have special team colours.

KID STUFF

Children stay fit because the games they like to play demand a lot of energy. Just think about a simple thing like throwing a ball and running after it – for most of us that would constitute a lot of our weekly exercise! In fact if we joined in our children's games more often we wouldn't have to worry so much about getting into shape. Here are a few old enjoyable games, mostly played in teams but all sufficiently adaptable to suit everyone.

TUG OF WAR
Easy to organize but pretty strenuous. To do it properly you need two teams of eight plus a non-active 'captain' for each side who tells you when to heave and when to rest. Each team pulls on one end of a rope against the other side, the idea being to pull your opponents across a dividing line, down the middle of the area.

Contests are generally the best two out of three pulls. Done properly it can help to develop great strength. But it's easily adapted to suit all the family. See that each team is evenly matched as far as weight and strength are concerned.

FRENCH CRICKET
Makes good fielding practice for the real thing and it's a lot of fun for all the family, including Grandpa, as it's not too strenuous. Any number can play but it's best to have at least six of you. Usually it's played in teams but you can just have a straight competition between each other if you prefer. You need something to bat with – a tennis racket, cricket bat or just a stick and a rubber ball.

Each member of the team has a go at batting in turn. Stand with your heels together and defend your legs with the bat. You don't actually have to run anywhere to score – just swing the bat from hand to hand round your body, the complete circle giving you one run. If you move your feet you're out. Anyone who picks up the ball after you've hit it can throw it at you from any angle, aiming at your legs. Alternatively he can throw it to another fielder so he can have a go instead.

ROUNDERS
There are lots of different versions you can adapt to suit the local conditions – on the beach or in the garden. Normally you need four 'bases' in a circle, a bat and as you're playing for fun, a soft ball. There are two teams and someone throws the ball at the batsman who must hit it and then run like mad from base to base, scoring a rounder when making the full circle.

TAG BALL
Another old favourite. You can play it with any large soft ball. One of you must go after the ball while the others try to keep it by hitting it into the air or along the ground with their hands. When you actually get to touch the ball you then change places with the last person to play it.

LEAPFROG
We've all played it at some time. One child makes a 'leapfrog' back and another actually leaps over. But you can adapt it in a variety of ways, by playing in teams and having to jump over lots of backs, the first to make it being the winner.

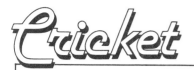

Cricket

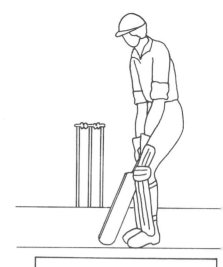

ON A STICKY WICKET

It's certainly not the fastest game around but it's a way of life in England, and the Commonwealth, part of the establishment where something that's 'not cricket' is bound to offend.

You play cricket in two teams, each with eleven players, and you take it in turn to bat and field. And the object of the fielding side is obviously to get the batting side out as quickly as possible. On the other hand the batting team want to get as many runs as they can.

It's not an amazingly energetic game; it is possible to score runs without actually having to run anywhere. If the batsman hits the ball far enough past the boundary line round the ground he gets four runs just like that, and six if it crosses the line without bouncing.

Games can go on endlessly and first class cricket matches last for three six-hour days or even longer, but there are shorter matches, where the time is deliberately limited. There's a lot of sitting about in the 'pavilion' while you wait your turn to bat and even when the big moment comes you won't burn up masses of calories ... only 50 or 55 for ten minutes' play. Of course, local teams are often more energetic, and if you and your children are out there batting away, and running up and down, you can use up a lot of energy — and calories.

SPECIAL THOUGHTS ON CRICKET

Interestingly, even the expression 'hat trick' dates back to the days when cricketers wore top hats and any player who took three wickets with three successive balls was presented with a white top hat. Now he's usually given the ball instead.

● Cricket balls can be lethal. It makes sense only to use them under proper conditions. If you're just having a bit of fun in the garden use a softer ball.

WHAT YOU NEED, WHERE TO GO, HOW TO LEARN

● Normally you wear white; flannel trousers, a shirt, and a sweater for when it's chilly and sports shoes. You obviously need a bat — no more than $4\frac{1}{2}$ inches wide and 38 inches long. When you are batting you'll need protective leg pads, and gloves. Most local teams have extra equipment for beginners.

● if your school has a team or any kind of club. Some towns and villages have a cricket team; they are almost always anxious to have new members, even beginners or out-of-condition, very elderly schoolboys the weekends; they are almost always anxious to have new members, even beginners or out-of-condition men who haven't played since school.

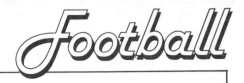

A FEW VARIATIONS

Canadian Football is almost like the American game, but the field is a little larger, and there are 12 men a side. Scoring is a little different, too, and penalties have different regulations, but basically it is a very similar game.

Australian Rules Football is quite different; played on an oval pitch, 18 players try to score through a pair of posts at opposite sides. The players are dressed simply in jerseys and shorts, the ball may be kicked or punched around, but not thrown, and the game is fast, furious, but not nearly as brutal as American or Canadian football.

AMERICAN FOOTBALL

Possibly second only to baseball, football is the most popular team sport in the United States. High Schools and Universities take it very seriously, and good young players are sought after by even exclusive colleges.

The game itself is played 11-a-side, with an oval ball, and on a rectangular field 360' by 160' wide. The actual playing area is marked off every five yards by chalk lines and it's divided into two sides, or zones, for the opposing teams. A team scores by carrying the ball into the opponent's zone, and they advance the ball by running with it, or by passing in a series of sometimes complicated team plays. The opposition recovers possession by blocking, tackling, and pulling down the ball carrier. A game is theoretically one hour long with breaks every 15 minutes, and the highest score wins. Very much a male game, there are very few mixed teams because of the hard physical contact. Children love football of all kinds and it is first-class exercise for them, and very strong on team spirit. It will burn up around 100 calories in 10 minutes play.

TOUCH FOOTBALL

Touch football is much less strenuous than ordinary football, there is no tackling, and touching the ball carrier is enough to indicate a 'down'. Families and friends out for the day or the afternoon often prefer touch football because it is easier on the players.

WHAT YOU NEED, WHERE TO GO, HOW TO LEARN

- Protective gear is the most important clothing; helmet and face mask, shoulder, pelvis and knee padding make ordinary men look like hulking giants. Jerseys, knee pants, socks and cleated shoes complete the uniform.

- Touch football can be played in casual loose clothing and canvas shoes with rubber soles.

- Find an existing team through a school, YMCA or health club.

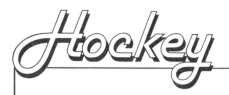

FIELD HOCKEY

These days it's quite a 'nice' game, part of the standard subjects for many hearty schoolgirls. That's why its origins are so interesting. For there was nothing nice about the Irish hurling as played in ancient times and it's thought that hockey developed from it. One record has the story of a truly lethal match in which the losing team also lost their lives.

When hockey first started, it had no refinements. The stick with which you hit the ball was often used to hit the opposition. Today it's played on a field, with eleven players to a side, positioned rather like a football team. Instead of kicking, they have a small white ball which is hit with the special flat wooden stick curving up at one end. The game is normally divided into two halves, each lasting 35 minutes and the idea is to score goals by driving the ball over your opposing team's goal line. It's a pretty good all-round fitness sport, especially for agility, building up muscles and stamina.

Most schools have hockey teams and there are national and Olympic teams, too. Mixed hockey, by the way, is very popular.

BEFORE YOU BEGIN

● Be careful how you wave your stick about; it *is* dangerous.

● Hockey is basically a game for young people.

● Shinguards are usually required and are very important. Most organized teams will supply them.

WHAT YOU NEED, WHERE TO GO, HOW TO LEARN

● A regular hockey stick ... try out several weights until you get one that's right for you but it mustn't be more than 28 ounces.

● Clothes should be loose and comfortable. Shorts and shirt are fine. Normally the club or team you join will have special gear including long hockey socks, shinguards and safety equipment.

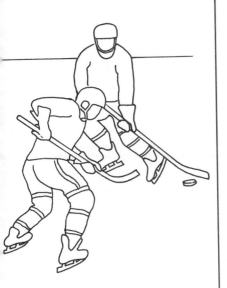

ICE HOCKEY

Back in 1860, the first game of ice hockey was played by the men of a Royal Canadian Rifles regiment in Kingston, Ontario. Today it's one of the biggest spectator sports, especially in Canada.

Ice hockey is incredibly fast. It is played with six on a team. The rink measures 200 feet by 85 feet. A rubber puck or disc is hit along the ice with a specially shaped wooden stick. Each game is divided into three rounds of twenty minutes each and there are normally between 11 and 18 players in each team as substitutes are often used.

There's a goalkeeper or 'goalie', three forwards and two defence men. The second most important thing to master is handling the stick without tripping yourself up, or fouling your opponents. Of course, the primary object is to shoot the puck into the opponents' goal.

As exercise, it's good for developing stamina and muscles but where ice hockey really scores is fast co-ordination of movement. It's good return for the energy you put in, burning up over 200 calories in just ten minutes play.

Understandably, it's basically a young person's sport and for a fit young person at that. It's a rough game, but many girls are joining teams.

WORTH NOTING

Some schools and universities with sports complexes have ice hockey rinks open to the public at specified times. Always play at a rink, never on a lake or river.

WHAT YOU NEED, WHERE TO GO, HOW TO LEARN

● You *must* wear the proper clothing. Shoulder guards, elbow and knee pads, shin guards, thick gauntlet-type gloves and generally a special helmet are required. Goalies must have even more protection including face masks. Most rinks which cater to ice hockey teams have equipment for hire and some coaching available. Lessons are vital to start with, then practice makes perfect.

● You'll need to buy or hire skates with ankle supports, reinforced caps at toe and heel, plus moulded arch support and tendon protector.

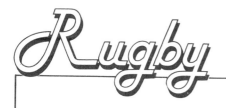

RUGBY UNION

Rugby Union is an amateur game, played in many countries, but it's especially popular in the UK and the Commonwealth.

Rugby is played with 15 men on a side, with an oval ball. The object is to score by getting the ball across your opponent's line, at the end of the field, or kicking it over the crossbar of the H-shaped goal posts.

The rules are quite complicated; play can get quite rough, especially in the scrummage, and no protective clothing is worn.

It's not really suitable for mixed teams, but men who have played rugby at school can go on playing reasonably well for quite a while as long as they are fit and used to considerable exercise. Rugby is quite a good burner of calories – the average player will use up 100 calories for every ten minutes' play. It's good exercise, although you may end up a little black and blue, since shouldering a player with the ball is allowed, and there are fewer penalities for rough handling than in soccer. Of course, intentional fouling is always penalized.

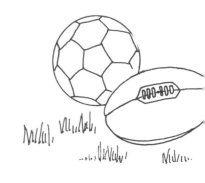

RUGBY LEAGUE

Rugby League is the professional form of Rugby which developed from Union rules. There are now many variations, and playing techniques are different, too. There are 13 men instead of 15 and it's played all around the world.

WHAT YOU NEED, WHERE TO GO, HOW TO LEARN

- Rugby clothing is simple – a pair of loose shorts and a jersey shirt are all that is necessary, although shin guards may be worn, too. Boots are usually required for team players.

- The ball is slightly rounded, but an oval football could be used in an emergency.

- Rugby must be played on a field or in the park – there is too much scrummaging and possible injury for hard-surfaced areas.

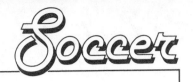

SOCCER, OR ASSOCIATION FOOTBALL

Soccer had been an English and European sport for years, but today it has become one of the most popular team games in countries all over the world. More and more amateur teams are also discovering that soccer is quick, enjoyable, and wonderful exercise for all the players.

The field is 100 yards by 50 yards, the ball is round, and the object is to get the ball into the goal defended by the opposing team. No player, with the exception of the goalkeeper in front of the net goal cage, can touch the ball with his hands. Players usually kick or 'head' the ball, although it can be propelled by any part of the body as long as it is not handled. Opponents regain possession of the ball by intercepting passes, or by tackling a player with the feet. Any kicking, pushing, tripping or charging is a foul.

The good thing about soccer is that anyone can play, you don't really need any special equipment except the ball – even a beach ball will do. Mixed teams can be made up although it's a good idea to keep an even distribution of men, women and children on both sides. It's a year-round game, playable even in the snow, although ice can be dangerous.

Soccer is athletic and strenuous, but not dependent on brute strength. Running builds up leg muscles, and you'll use up around 90 calories in ten minutes. It's a really first-class family game for Sunday afternoon with friends.

ANY PLACE, ANY WHERE

One of the good things about soccer is its adaptability. You can play on a field, in the park, even on a quiet street closed to traffic – the only requirement is that both the goals at opposite ends are the same width. Use chalk marks.

WHAT YOU NEED, WHERE TO GO, HOW TO LEARN

• Clothing is optional except when you play on a recognized team. Normally loose, casual shorts and a shirt would be fine, with canvas or leather rubber-soled shoes to run and kick in. Nothing that causes injury should be worn – that means rings, belt buckles, scarves or hard shoes.

• A ball is all the equipment that is necessary.

• There are many local teams in offices, YMCA's and sports clubs, and many schools encourage outside teams to play their students.

Volleyball and Netball

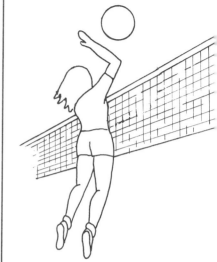

VOLLEYBALL

In 1895 William Morgan in Massachusetts was worried about encouraging middle-aged businessmen to come to his gym for exercise, so he invented volleyball as the perfect sport for mixed age groups with very mixed abilities.

It's a team game, played indoors on a special court, or on any flat bit of grass – there's a high net across the middle of a rectangle, roughly 30 by 60 feet, with six players on a side, volleying the large, inflated ball across the net using hands.

A point is scored everytime the ball touches the ground on the opposing side before they have a chance to return it. Three players on each side can help the ball on its way, then it must be sent across the net. Only the serving team can score, a set means a minimum of fifteen points scored, with a two-point lead, and a match is the best of three or five sets. An important part of the game is rotating positions, which gives everyone on the team a chance at different strokes, and a chance to serve, too. Volleyball isn't violent exercise – only burning up around 50 calories for every ten minutes of play, but it does help flexibility and quick movement, and it is first-class physical recreation. But remember if you haven't played regularly it can be strenuous to keep waving your arms in the air as you reach for the ball, so take it easy and don't play for too long.

WHAT YOU NEED, WHERE TO GO, HOW TO LEARN

● Shorts, a tea shirt and tennis or non-slip shoes are the best clothes, with a sweater to put on if it gets chilly outdoors.

● A volleyball net is set about eight feet high, with posts. In a gym this is always provided, but if you and your neighbours really enjoy it, you can use two convenient trees, or ordinary stakes, and buy the net – if the team chips i⬤ it's not expensive at all.

NETBALL

Netball is similar to basketball, but with seven players on each team who are restricted to certain areas of the court and it is sometimes played outdoors. The net doesn't have a backboard, although it's the same height as the basketball net. Players may throw the ball, or pass it, but they cannot run with it as basketball players do. Netball is usually played by girls and women.

**SPECIAL NOTE FOR
FAMILY OR BUSINESS OUTINGS:**

Volleyball's especially good for group outings like family picnics or company meetings, because people of very mixed abilities can play easily together. Don't get too bogged down in the finer points, just encourage everybody to get up and play – children enjoy it enormously because the ball is fairly light, and easy to volley. Never use a heavy ball – it can be very painful and sprain your wrist or hit someone on the head.

● You must use a real volleyball. In an emergency, a beachball is the only useful alternative, but it may be too light to serve properly.

● Get a schoolteacher or a local enthusiast to give you the basic instruction – it's not difficult to learn, and it's definitely more fun to do than just to sit around and to watch.

● A netball ring is set about 10 feet high; you can use a basketball ring in an emergency.

Looking Good

Introduction

GOOD LOOKS, GOOD LIVING, FROM TOP TO TOE

Getting healthy and feeling fit also means looking naturally good, caring for yourself in every possible way. Just in case you think that taking pains to look well is pure vanity, think again. Your appearance and how you look after yourself reflects your whole life. Sloppy and careless? Chances are you are not making the most of your potential in other areas of your life. If you treat yourself with real respect, then this healthy self-awareness will reflect in your work, play, and in your relationships with other people. The rock bottom of any daily routine is cleanliness – something that is particularly important in the development of children's self-esteem. When a troubled child's self-confidence improves, so does an interest in physical appearance, and the time and care put into being attractive . After they learn the delights of bathtime, with boats or plastic ducks or bubble bath, the chances are you won't be able to keep the once water-shy creature out of the bathroom. The next problem is how to get the bathtub cleaned up with the same interest … but that's another story.

In recent years we have sometimes carried a passion for washing perhaps further than it need be. In every respect of health and fitness and all our lives the right balance is essential. There is every reason to enjoy the fresh scent of cleanliness, but that doesn't mean tons of lather spread lavishly over the skin, or two to three baths a day, plus a line-up of bottles more suitable for a supermarket shelf than a bathroom cabinet.

Hair dyes, deodorants, toothpaste, feminine deodorants, shaving soaps, mouth-washes, foot powders, douches, setting lotions, hair sprays, air fresheners, household soaps and detergents, make-up, household cleaners etc. – how many and how much do we really need?

One of the most important myths to explode is the ideal of germ-free people in an antiseptic household. Of course, harmful bacteria are responsible for the growth of infections and diseases. And no one is suggesting we should live in filthy homes piled high with dirt, breeding grounds of disintegrating food and unpleasant rubbish.

But most of us live today in reasonable comfort, and keep a reasonable standard of cleanliness. We mustn't be frightened into being nervous wrecks, stalking the germs through cracks and crannies, pouring disinfectant everywhere, ashamed if a neighbour spots a film of dust or a stray footmark on a shiny, squeaky-clean floor!

In the first place, there is no such thing as a germ-free household, and a good thing too. When animals and/or people are kept in a completely germ-free atmosphere, they become over-susceptible to infection. Take them out of their artificially-pure environment, and they rapidly get all sorts of minor – and sometimes major – illnesses. Basically it is vital for healthy people to live in a normal atmosphere where they are subject to a reasonable level of bacteria in their day-to-day lives; it helps develop resistance to disease, and build up a solid level of tolerance for normal life. We are not hot-house flowers, and we are all the healthier for it!

So stop worrying and start enjoying your housework, and your body. Polish the furniture when it needs doing, not every time a fingermark appears, and use a lemon or lavender scented mild polish. Treat yourself in the same way – use a mild, scented soap, enjoy pampering yourself, don't think you need to be covered in creams and sprays to be attractive. Brush your hair, but not too hard, clean your skin, but don't scrub away the protective layers. Take pride in your home, and in yourself as you go through daily routines. Let your mind relax – you're worth paying attention to! When you are completely involved in what you are doing, the doing itself takes you far from anxiety and tension.

Caring for yourself is another part of fitness, along with good nutrition, relaxation and exercise. You need a springboard to help you jump off into real living and working. Look in the mirror, and like what you see – there you are, looking good!

THE MAGIC OF MASSAGE

Massage can tone you up and calm you down, relieve aching muscles and help you when you feel tired or under stress. There are hundreds of books on massage and how to do it, but you don't need any special movements nor do you have to memorize lists of techniques to do it well. Every good masseur has his own style and way of treating the muscles. You can also develop your own simply by practice.

Massage yourself when you get out of the bath, or your husband or wife when aching muscles need rest. It is also great used on children who have trouble settling down for the night. There is something quite magical about touching another body with awareness. A form of non-verbal communication takes place that can be soothing and healing for both of you.

Get yourself a bottle of baby oil. Start on the back, moving gently but firmly up the sides of the spine with the palms of your hands and down again, then put pressure on the spine itself. The more you relax into it, the more you will find your hands make their own natural movements as they knead, stroke, soothe the body. It takes a little bit of practice but soon it will all start to fall into place. For the face, use the tips of your fingers and palms of your hands. Then go on to the area at the base of the head and the shoulders where tension tends to lock itself in chronically. Do the spine again, concentrating particularly on the sacral area at the base, then go on to the arms and legs. The more you enjoy your work the better your skill in massage will become, and you'll discover the delight of massaging and being massaged.

WHEN NATURE NEEDS A LITTLE HELP

Everybody needs a little pampering … a soothing bath after a long day, the gentle massage of tense and tired muscles, an occasional sauna, a brisk rub-down with a loofah to get rid of old dead skin. But few people pamper themselves enough. Partly this is because of long-standing puritanical attitudes that make any attention you pay to yourself seem slightly shameful. Mostly it is just simple neglect. We get involved in other responsibilities, and don't think about our own needs. All very well until a pulled aching muscle or continual tiredness makes you stop in your tracks and demand that you do something.

Here is a practical list of treatments and recipes to use every now and then whenever you need them, or whenever you have enough time to indulge yourself. In terms of lasting health and fitness the time you spend will never be wasted.

For nature lovers, try a lavender water made up of 6 drops of pure oil of lavender in a pint of distilled water. Store in a dark bottle, keep in the refrigerator and apply twice a day with a clean pad to the parts of the body that perspire easily.
Or use green leaves, green vegetable tops, or fresh herbs such as mint, rubbing briskly under the arms (chlorophyll is a natural deodorant, as air freshener manufacturers know well).

BATH AND WATER TREATMENTS

Take a lavender bath when you're strung up. Add a few drops of essential oil of lavender to the bath water to relax body and mind. Soak for 15 minutes.

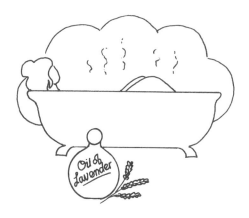

Take a variable temperature bath when you're worn out. Run a bath of hot water and lie down to soak. When you're relaxed, turn on the cold tap so it runs slowly into the tub, gradually cooling down the temperature. When the water drops below body temperature, get out, dry yourself briskly and dress warmly. This is ideal after a long exhausting day to revive you for a full evening ahead.

Make an Oatmeal Bag. Fill a little muslin bag, about 4" × 6", with raw oatmeal and tie the open end with a piece of string. Use it in the bath to rub all over the body. The paste from the grain smoothes and softens skin. Ideal for dry parched legs and arms after exposure to the sun. A bag can be used several times before changing the oatmeal again.

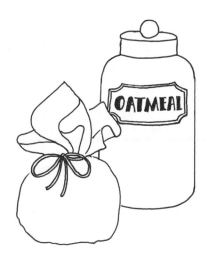

Take a sauna when you need relief from mental and physical tension. The warmth and the rise in your body temperature eases mental and bodily tensions by relaxing muscles all over. Sweating also eliminates wastes that can build up in the system and leaves skin smooth and glowing. An ideal way to relax after exercise. The only people who need to steer clear of saunas are those with high or low blood pressure, heart disease, pregnant mothers and people on very strict diets. Be sure to lie down and rest for half an hour after a sauna to give your body a chance to return to normal.

Discover the benefits of a hemp glove and use it daily. Rub over the surface of the body briskly for five minutes before a bath or shower. This has an immediate beneficial action on the muscles, stimulates circulation, removes the dead layers of cells from the surface of the skin, and helps to smooth out the fatty lumps and bumps that can appear on the thighs of even the slimmest women.

Jump into a cold shower. It will do wonders to wake you up and get you going. Begin with a five minute hot shower. Then when the skin begins to glow with the warmth, make the water cold and stand under it for one minute. Get out, dry briskly and dress warmly.

SEE WHAT HERBS HAVE TO OFFER

Herb teas can help calm you down, pep you up, soothe a slightly upset tummy, get rid of excess fluids in the tissues. Experiment until you find what works best for you.

To make tea: Steep 2 tablespoons dried leaves or flowers in a pot of boiled water for five minutes.

Camomile: Soothes upset stomachs and calms jangled nerves.

Mint: A mild stimulant. Good too for dyspepsia and flatulence.

Golden Rod and Nettle: Excellent for helping to get rid of excess fluid that can make you feel waterlogged and clog tissues of thighs and hips.

Goldenseal, Skullcap, Valerian: Nerve tonics and internal cleansers. Good for unwinding when under excess strain, and as a nightcap before bed.

Posture and Presence

STANDING TALL

How you stand, sit, move, hold, and carry yourself affects fitness on so many levels it is difficult to list them all. Yet few people today have what can be called *good* posture – the correct relationship between the head and the vertebrae of the spine. Being too fat, or the wrong way of standing, sitting, lifting and moving can be a direct cause of leg and back aches, disc troubles, faulty co-ordination of muscles, and fatigue. Or they can even result in faulty breathing, strain and feelings of depression, boredom and indifference. Correct posture helps physical troubles and mental ones, too – your whole attitude towards yourself and your life usually changes for the better. The relationship between good posture and overall fitness is fundamental.

The spine is made up of a series of natural curves which offer the body good balance, and support all its movements. When the spine remains strong and healthy, these curves are responsible for helping the body to stay in the most comfortable position. Between each separate vertebra in the spinal column is a pad or cushion of cartilage with a soft core known as vertebral disc. These discs act like shock absorbers, protecting the vertebrae from being damaged by a sudden movement, the impact of running or jumping and so forth. When the back has to bear an unusual or sudden strain, one of the soft cores may begin to protrude slightly from the edges of the vertebrae and you get the very unpleasant pain of a herniated disc.

The strength and support for all the vertebrae in the spinal column comes from a highly complex system of muscles that spans the back. When these muscles are strong, flexible and resilient, then the back they support can usually take any number of movements without damage. When they become shortened, weak, or restricted in their movements, the back becomes highly vulnerable to damage and pain. This is why regular practice of exercises for flexibility is vital, especially as we get older, and all our muscles weaken. The other cause of much back trouble is misuse. When you stoop to lift something, you may bend the spine instead of bending the large hip joint and knee joint and taking the strain in the legs. Such a poor practice causes aches and damage to musculature and bones in the back. In addition, using your spine instead of your legs means you can't lift anywhere near the weight you are capable of carrying.

Posture affects how you look too. If the natural curve in the lower spine is too great, your pelvis will be tilted too much, your abdomen will stick out and your chest will sink in, making you look shorter and a lot heavier than you are. The secret of good posture is simple and far from the old school directives to pull your stomach in and force your shoulders back. (This kind of military stance can do as much harm as the sloppy-joe slouch.) Forcing the shoulders back unnaturally leads to tension in the muscles of the shoulder girdle that result in stiffness and pain; pushing the chest out, along with the sucked-in abdomen, prevents the full movement of the ribs and restricts breathing. Pulling your stomach in, though, is generally good, provided your back is flat, and the buttocks tucked in.

Here's how to get it right. If you imagine youself being suspended from the ceiling by a fine cord that passes through your head, and down the middle of your spine, you will feel the natural alignment of your body. The limbs and shoulders come out from this central column and hang freely from it, so they can move easily. When you get this right, everything else will fall naturally into place, too. Your feet will be in line just off parallel and your weight supported evenly over the whole surface of the feet (high heel wearers take note. Stiletto heels may make your legs look great but they do nothing for your posture at all.) Legs will be straight but not braced and arms will hang freely from the shoulders. Rather awkward at first, but once you get the right balance you will begin to feel different – lighter, freer in your movements and even more peaceful.

Whenever you find yourself becoming tense during the day, it is a good idea to stop and 're-align things'; it can have a remarkably refreshing effect on all of you. You won't suffer as much from fatigue. And as the years go by, good habits of posture will keep you free of so many of the unpleasant aches and pains which are usually associated with age but which are far more likely to be the result of postural neglect.

Form good habits for sitting, standing, lifting and sleeping and they will pay you endless dividends in mobility and a trouble-free back, not to mention what they can do for your physical presence when you come into a room. Good posture gives an impression of vitality, confidence and health that will keep you attractive for life. It not only protects against damage, it also lends a natural grace to ordinary movements.

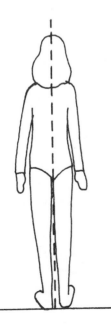

The right way to sit

Choose a chair with a high back that offers support to the lower spine. As you sit, lower yourself into the chair (instead of flopping down), bending at the hips and knees and keeping your back as straight as possible. Put your feet on the floor a few inches apart for support and let your arms and shoulders hang freely from a well supported, erect spine. When you are sewing or working with your hands or reading, in a chair, bring the object of your attention up near your face instead of bending your back to bring your face down to it.

The right way to lift

Never bend from the waist; it puts far too much strain on the back muscles and not enough on your legs which are stronger and more capable of taking it. Instead, keep your back straight, and bending from the knees and the large hip joint, squat to get under the package you are going to lift. Then, back still straight, lift with the muscles of your legs gradually straightening up and automatically lifting the package as you do so.

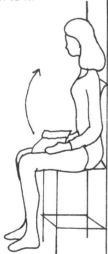

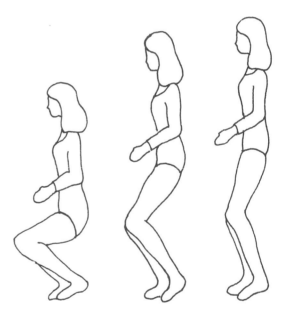

The right way to sleep

Choose a good firm mattress that gives support to the whole spine so there is no danger of hanging on to residual tension in the muscles (this can happen on a bed that's too soft) or putting too much of any curve in the spine and letting it bend unnaturally in sleep. A piece of hardboard under a soft mattress will do the trick. You might feel a bit stiff for the first couple of nights if you have been used to a soft bed but the stiffness will soon pass and your spine will benefit immeasurably from the change. It's better to throw away a mattress that's losing its firmness and buy a new one than wait until it wears out. The expense will be more than justified by trouble-free backs.

The right way to carry

When you have shopping to carry, distribute it evenly between two bags, taking one in each hand to avoid straining one side of the body. Carry them freely, allowing the shoulders to take the load. There is no need to tense up the shoulder muscles, either. This will only lead to early fatigue.

The right way to work standing

If you have to lean over a sink or work bench, bend your knees to bring yourself down to the proper level instead of stooping at the shoulders. (Stooping can lead to aches in the upper back and neck, fatigue and mid-back pain.)

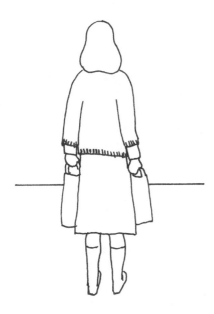

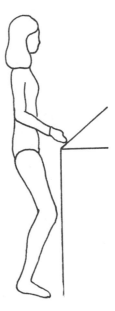

Whenever you have been using your shoulder muscles for a long time, try to relax them even for just a few minutes. Put down the shopping, and do the little exercise on page 270. You'll find the break really makes a difference.

If you must bend over straighten up every few minutes, or better still, move away from your work, and swing your arms over your head and around in a windmill.

For long standing periods, use a small stool to put up one foot for a few minutes. It breaks the tension and relaxes the calf muscles.

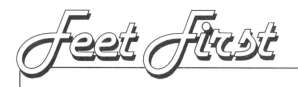

AT THE FOOT OF FITNESS

Feet matter. When they are healthy they help keep you full of bounce and free from physical strain. When they ache, you can feel irritable, tense and strained, and end up with premature lines even on a young face. If they are imprisoned day after day in ill-fitting shoes they contribute to the development of circulatory problems such as varicose veins, and to backache, putting unnatural strain on many of the body's important systems. Cramped and uncomfortable feet can even interfere with digestive processes. Obesity can also cause a lot of trouble for feet. And feeling tired all the time may be caused by a foot problem. Mobility can be a real difficulty, especially with older people. When painful feet or neglected bunions make walking difficult, it seems easier to sit or lie down more and more of the time. Gradually the whole lung and heart system slows down, and then deteriorates rapidly. If even a mild heart attack occurs, there may not be enough reserve in the system to cope with the loss of power, and recovery is terribly slow, and not always sure.

Little wonder feet are important. No part of your body is subjected to such constant pressure and use. Each foot is made up of 26 delicate little bones bound together with powerful muscles and ligaments that hold them in place.

They are enormously complex mechanisms designed to take a combined load of more than a million pounds as we walk an average of several miles on them each day. Unfortunately, they are also neglected and abused because few people realise what a profound effect feet can have on their general health.

About 90 per cent of all troubles come from ill-fitting shoes – heels that are too high, toes that are too pointed, too narrow or just the wrong shape. And every foot has its own special curves that have to be taken into account when chosing a pair of shoes. For instance, not only is width and length important, but so is the distance between the heel and the metatarsal arch, and the length of the toes. All of these measurements depend on the *last* of the shoe (the specific form around which a shoe has been built or made). Usually there are two or three lasts that will suit each person's feet. Shop carefully those that are really comfortable and then stick to them, buying your shoes from the same manufacturer so you can be sure of getting a standard size and shape.

In choosing a shoe there are several important things to look for: First, is it wide enough and long enough? Your toes should never touch the end, and you should be able to take a small pinch in the leather across the widest part of the shoe to ensure that there is 'leeway'. Then, does it give good support under the instep with room for your foot to spread inside the shoe? Cramping leads to deformities such as ingrown nails, bunions, and corns. Make sure you try both left and right shoes – most of us have one larger foot. Choose the larger shoe size, and have a pad or extra sole fitted for the smaller foot.

Is the heel height right? Too high a heel (above 2'' to 2$\frac{1}{2}$''), holds the foot rigid when you walk instead of allowing it to bend freely with each step. This bending and stretching movement is essential for proper circulation, not only in the feet themselves but also in the legs. It exercises the muscles of the lower extremities as you move, keeping muscles toned and blood vessels strong and clear. Too low a heel can lead to aches in your calves.

To find your ideal heel height, sit in a chair, legs crossed, so one leg hangs freely and the foot attached to it is relaxed. Now place a straight flat surface, such as a card along its length, flat against the ball of the foot and extending beyond the heel. Measure the distance between the bottom of your heel and the card beneath it with a ruler and you have the ideal heel height for you. Choose your shoes as much as possible to correspond to this measurement.

shoe that a child wears, takes on the particular individual imprint of his foot. So shoes should never be passed on to a younger child. Going barefoot is one of the best things you can do for your feet and legs; try to do it often. These things can make all the difference between foot health and foot trouble. Dealing with foot troubles after they have developed can be very complicated, while looking after your feet is easy and reaps immeasurable benefits in good looks, good health and high spirits.

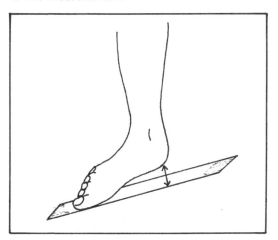

If you are buying shoes for young children remember that they should be fitted for width and length every couple of months. Each

FOOT PROBLEMS AND HOW TO DEAL WITH THEM

Rough skin and callouses

Try spreading petroleum jelly thickly on the roughened area then covering it with a cotton sock for the night. In the morning use one of the callous removers, a liquid lotion that you spread on and rub in while it rubs off the dead skin. It may take two or three treatments to get rid of the hardness, if your feet have been neglected.

Corns

They come from friction or pressure, the skin's natural attempt to protect itself. Corns form a heavy thick protective cone-shaped layer, with the point, or eye of the cone at the deepest level on the inside. If the eye presses against a nerve this can cause severe pain. The only way to get rid of corns is by professional treatment. Cutting them out yourself can be dangerous and lead to infection. But you can soak them in hot salt water for 20 minutes for temporary relief then wear a padded ring around the area to eliminate pressure.

Bunions

This hard swelling at the base of the big toe comes from poor fitting shoes that cause the big toe to bend inwards and the base of the toe to stick out to the side. At the first sign, see a specialist. He will treat it and give you special exercises to correct the problem plus a pad of lint or rubber to wear for protection inside shoes. If the bunion is too developed surgery may be the only answer.

Plantar Warts

Sometimes called verrucas, these painful spots are the result of a virus infection, usually picked up from walking barefoot in public places such as swimming pools or school gyms. They appear either singly or in groups, and if mild can sometimes clear up themselves. But because they grow inwards, they can cause a lot of pain. If they don't clear up spontaneously they will need medical treatment either by electrical burning, freezing, or the use of acid pastes or liquids. Surgery is necessary if the wart is too deeply embedded in the foot.

Nail fungus

Called onychomicosis, the problem is caused by a fungus that attacks the nail, making it discolour and thicken so much that it is difficult or impossible to cut or clip. The fungus can easily spread, and thrives in a warm dark condition, so feet should be kept clean and dry. A liquid fungicide is painted underneath the nail and the edge gradually clipped away. The cure can take weeks to complete but requires only a few moments a day for treatment.

Ingrown toenails

Caused by wrong clipping of the nail (clipping in a curve rather than straight across) or by shoes that are too tight, this can be a terribly painful problem and requires professional advice. Don't leave it. If it is mistreated or ignored the problem can be there for life.

Athlete's foot

This common problem is caused by a highly contagious fungus and is best treated by avoiding the things that can bring it on in the first place. In other words, keep feet dry and cool, clean, stay away from infected people and from contact with the floors of changing rooms in public swimming pools and gyms. The signs are flaking or splitting of the skin, often between the toes, an itchy rash and even blisters on the bottom of toes and feet. Treat it by rubbing away dead skin with a pumice stone and applying a preparation designed to kill the fungus. Keep the stone you use apart, and sterilize it after every use in a bowl of disinfectant and water. Expose your feet to the air as much as possible and use a special fungicidal dusting powder. Be sure to change stockings and socks regularly and dry well between the toes after washing feet or taking a bath or shower.

HOW TO LOOK AFTER YOUR FEET

- Wash feet every day with a stiff brush, part by part. Use a pumice stone to get rid of any callouses or rough spots.

- Dust your feet with foot powder, especially if they tend to perspire freely. This helps dry them out and prevents smells.

- Always cut your toenails straight across with a scissors or special toenail clipper. This helps prevent ingrown toenails.

- Change socks, nylons and tights at least once a day. Make sure both shoes and socks are the right size. Even socks and stockings that are too small can cause foot problems by restricting movement in the toes.

- If a foot problem develops, don't ignore it. Instead go to a chiropodist for treatment. Difficulties dealt with when they first appear are easy to treat. Left until later, they can lead to compound problems.

SPECIAL TREATS AND TREATMENTS

Aching feet
Give them an Epsom salts bath: mix three tablespoons of salts to a quart of warm water. Plunge your feet first into salt bath for five minutes, then into ice cold water for 30 seconds. Then prop them up above your head against a wall or held up by a cushion for 10 minutes.

Sweating feet
Plunge them into a lukewarm bath to which you've added a few drops of oil of lavender, and let them soak for five minutes.

Quick relief
Spray with cologne and change your stockings or socks.

Standing all day
Carry an extra pair of shoes with you and change the height of your heels a few times throughout the day.

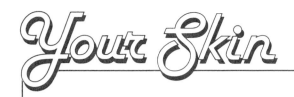

MORE THAN A COVERING FOR YOUR BODY

Your skin is far more than just the decorative outside layer of your body. It is its largest organ, covering an area of between 15 and 20 square feet, accounting for about 16 per cent of your weight, and reflecting the condition of your whole system. Few skin problems are only skin deep!

The outer skin is made up of two layers, the epidermis, or outer covering, and the dermis, or true skin, with the sweat glands, nerves and capillaries that nourish the cells of both layers. The skin is elastically attached to the underlying tissues of muscles which gives it flexibility, and a beautifully firm and spongy feel. With age, the skin loses its natural padding and resilance, and sagging and wrinkling take place.

This complex organ, has important jobs to perform protecting the delicate internal organs and tissues, acting as a barrier against physical damage, bacterial infection and the sun's harmful ultra-violet rays. It is also our finest sensory organ, so that we have immediate sensations of pain, pleasure, heat and cold and providing the nervous system and brain with a continuous flow of information about the environment. Skin also regulates the body's temperature and is responsible for 85 per cent of its heat loss. When your body is exposed to heat from hot weather or a hot bath, the little capillaries near its surface dilate to allow greater blood flow through them and greater heat loss outwards into the air. Body heat is also lost through the skin by perspiration, one and a

half pints a day in a temperate zone. When it is cold outside, these vessels contract to reduce blood flow near the surface and conserve radiant energy. Finally, your skin can manufacture Vitamin D from exposure to the sun and even produce some important antibodies.

In short, skin is a living breathing thing that needs to be cared for, not treated as a superficial layer, ignored except when there are signs of trouble. Good skin-care will make you look glowing and vital as the years go by. How fast your skin ages depends more on its treatment and the general condition of your whole body than on age. Of course, genetic inheritance matters too. But apart from general unhealthiness, the three main culprits behind prematurely-aging skin are the sun, cigarettes and air pollution in that order.

We have become a society of sun-worshippers, the glorious golden tan is a symbol of freedom, status and leisure which we all want, sometimes at any cost. But the price we pay for it is often high in terms of prematurely aging skin and sagging contours. Ultra-violet rays stimulate certain cells in the skin to distribute a pigment called melanin; the same deadly light rays cause changes in the cells of the dermis, leading to rapid aging, sagging and wrinkled skin, and in cases of prolonged extreme exposure, to skin cancer.

Tanning is nothing more than a defence mechanism. The melanin that turns the skin brown is the only way the skin has of offering a protective layer to guard itself and the deeper layers of the body from ultra-violet damage. Certainly the damage done to skin cells and to the connective tissues is a great deal worse if the skin is allowed to burn. But even if the skin suffers no burning the damaging changes from exposure to sunlight still occur and so does premature aging. The damage may not show up immediately, until wrinkles appear several years later. To preserve youthful, healthy-looking skin, tan little (go for the pale golden look on your body instead of the baked skin à la St Tropez), and avoid the sun on your face altogether by using a good moisturiser complete with sunscreen, plus a high protection sunscreen that blocks all the ultra-violet rays. Use a lower protection product for your body and let it gently brown. Increase your exposure to the sun gradually, starting with 20 minutes a day (never between the hours of 11 a.m. and 3 p.m.) and stepping it up by 10 or 15 minutes each day until you build up a good protective tan.

Cigarettes, too, damage the skin. Dermatological tests show that smokers' skins appear 10 to 20 years older than those of non smokers. This is believed to be because each cigarette you smoke depletes your system of 25 milligrams of Vitamin C which is necessary for the health and strength of our tissues.

Looking after your skin is simple. Cleanliness comes first. But this doesn't mean scrubbing away with great volumes of soap that can clog pores and remove the skin's natural oils. Use soap sparingly and only in the places it is needed most — under the arms, around the genitals, and wherever you are actually dirty. On the face, use a neutral soap, a mild

detergent cleanser or a lotion cleanser that is pH balanced so that it doesn't remove the skin's natural acid mantle, which helps protect it from bacterial invasion and excessive drying. Be sure to remove any make-up completely and let your skin breathe by not covering it day and night with a heavy film of make-up or cream.

For both men and women, a moisturizer with a sunscreen is a good idea. Men can apply it after shaving in the morning. This helps protect against ultra-violet rays and excessive water loss from heat, dry air, or air-conditioning systems. Drying out can be another cause of prematurely aging skin.

Finally, to be sure your skin is getting everything it needs to stay healthy and glowing, eat plenty of raw fruits and vegetables, grain products and lean protein foods.

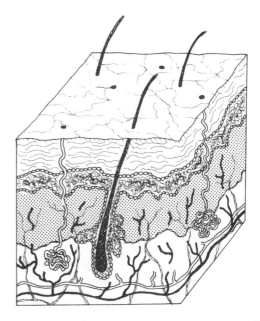

SKIN PROBLEMS AND HOW TO COPE WITH THEM

Blackheads

These are plugs of sebum or oil which clog the pores and blacken due to oxidation on exposure to the air. They can easily be removed if you take care not to damage the skin which could result in infection. Heat the skin first by applying a hot compress made of 1 tablespoon of bicarbonate of soda to a pint of hot water (as hot as your skin will take). Apply and re-apply the compress to the blackhead areas for about two minutes to open the pores and loosen the material clogging them. Then gently, with the tips of your fingers wrapped in a paper tissue, (*not* your nails) ease out the plug. Finish off with an application of alcohol or antiseptic cream.

Whiteheads

These are small, white, eruptions that never quite surface but remain as tiny beads under the outer layer of the skin. They are much like blackheads in their make-up but they don't turn black, as the matter trapped in the duct never reaches the surface and oxidises. A tiny opening has to be made in the centre of the bump with a sterile needle and the contents have to be eased out as in the case of blackheads.

Broken veins

Once there, they are impossible to get rid of except by a professional with the help of an electric needle or chemical injections which take several treatments over a period of time. The red veins are caused by fragility of tiny capillaries under the skin and can be prevented by avoiding extremes of temperature on the face (where they are most common) and by taking large quantities of extra Vitamin C – about 1500 mg a day plus the bioflavinoids which you can buy from a health-food store.

Warts

These are small, harmless growths on the skin which can be chemically removed or frozen with liquid oxygen. Many vanish without treatment. Any growth should be seen by the doctor at once.

Dermatitis

The term means inflamation of the skin and takes in such problems as eczema and psoriasis. Psoriasis is characterised by red patches and spots overlaid with loose, lighter scales. It usually affects the skin of elbows, legs, knees, arms and scalp. It is the result of too large a production of keratin (the outer scaly layers of the skin) but the original cause is unknown.

Eczema is the result of exposure to certain substances to which the body has a sensitivity (such as cosmetics, paints, detergents, metals aerosol sprays, etc) or comes as a result of emotional reactions. The blood vessels dilate and turn porous, which lets fluid from the cells of the skin collect and form blisters on the surface. They dry out and the area becomes itchy and encrusted, posing a serious threat of infection.

Both eczema and psoriasis can be treated dermatologically to clear up the symptoms but the real cure comes only from isolating the prime irritant and eliminating it.

Moles

These are raised brown areas and are made up of cells with a high concentration of melanin in them. They are usually harmless. They can be removed easily and painlessly by medical burning or surgery. Some are even considered beauty marks. If any mole should suddenly change in size or in any way, have it examined by your doctor at once.

Boils

These painful pus-filled bumps are the result of an infection of the hair follicle, a sweat gland, or a cut. They occur most often on someone who is generally run down and are often a way of the body eliminating toxic wastes from the system. Most boils literally heal themselves once the dead skin that makes up their core has been released. If there are many boils or they don't seem to clear up readily it is best to seek medical advice.

Bruising

Bruises are the result of small blood vessels that have been ruptured under the skin causing blood to seep into surrounding tissues and turning the area black and blue. As the blood is re-absorbed and the bruise heals they turn yellow or green until the area returns to normal.

In people who bruise regularly and too easily, the problem can often be helped by adding supplements of Vitamin C plus rutin and the bioflavoids to the diet. These vitamins are generally available in health-food stores and can be taken in amounts up to 2000 milligrams of Vitamin C daily without danger, as the vitamins are water soluble and any excess is readily eliminated from the body. In combination they help to strengthen the walls of the tiny blood vessles so they break less readily. Vitamin C on its own won't do the trick.

PERSPIRATION

It's a common mistake to imagine that perspiration causes the unpleasant body smell which all the advertisements warn us will keep even our best friends away. It doesn't. Perspiration itself is mostly clear water with a few mineral salts.

The eccrine glands are distributed evenly all over the body, responding to changes in outside temperature and physical exertion. If clothing, particularly synthetics, traps the water instead of letting it evaporate naturally, bacteria start to give off waste products which smell, and may also be absorbed into the clothing as stale sweat. The appocrine glands respond only to changes in emotion, they are under the arms, around the genitals, buttocks, and nipples. Their secretions are particularly attractive to the bacteria on the skin, so the largest amount of waste product will be given off in those areas. Anti-perspirants use chemicals to block the sweat ducts. Sometimes this causes unpleasant allergies, so try to use less by wearing mixtures of cotton, wool or silk, and applying either deodorant or anti-perspirant (or both in one product) only on a cool, dry skin. After a bath is *not* the best time – the skin is too damp, and the perspiration ducts are not open. Wait until you have cooled down, and your body is quiet.

Your Hair

THE CROWNING GLORY

The whole of your body – except for the palms of your hands and the soles of the feet – is covered with hair. It acts as a protection, conserves body heat by trapping air in spaces between hairs to insulate the skin and, in certain places, like the head, on a man's face and in the genital region. Hair plays a part in attracting the opposite sex. Perhaps this is why both men and women spend more time and money on their hair than on any other aspect of personal care.

On your head there are somewhere between 100,000 and 200,000 hairs at any one time. They grow on average half an inch a month in a regular cycle; a growth phase, followed by a rest phase, followed by a discard phase in which old hairs are pushed out by new hair growth from the scalp. You lose on average 100 hairs a day and get a whole new head of hair about every three years.

The thickness of your hair depends on the number of hair follicles you are born with, so does its coarseness or fineness, all of which are determined by heredity. Whether your hair is curly or straight depends on the curve of the follicles themselves. Straight hair comes from round follicles, wavy hair from kidney-shaped follicles and curly hair from very curved follicles. Within each follicle on the scalp is a sebaceous gland which secretes oil to keep hair pliable and sleek, a tiny muscle which makes hair both on the head and the body literally stand on end when you are frightened or cold and a system of capillaries that supply the follicles with nutrients from the blood stream.

The part of the hair we see, the hair itself, is called the shaft. It is made up of three important parts, the hollow central core, called the medulla, the middle layer called the cortex which gives the hair its colour and its elastic resilience, and an outer coating of keratin-based, scale-like cells that overlap each other and are known as the cuticle.

When the cuticle lies smooth and flat, it picks up and refracts the light, making the hair look shiny, gleaming and in good condition. When it is flaky and rough, a head of hair looks dull and lifeless. Conditioners smooth down the scales so that they lie flat and sleek. This also makes hair feel soft and smooth.

Diet and general health have a profound effect on your hair – how it looks and how it grows. Proteins, the B complex vitamins and many minerals, particularly iron, copper and iodine, are essential for strong healthy hair. The hair itself is made up mostly of protein, and protein and mineral deficiencies can be diagnosed in a laboratory simply by looking at a hair taken from the patient's head.

So although hair – like fingernails – is technically 'dead' not living tissue, it is closely linked to what is going on inside you – and really bad-looking hair may be a sign of poor general health and nutrition. Some hairdressers recommend taking nutritional supplements such as kelp tablets or a good B complex supplement. If your hair tends to be too greasy, try cutting down on oils and fats in your diet and cut out fried foods altogether. Drugs may also have unpleasant side effects on your hair – check with your doctor if you are taking any new medication.

HOW TO LOOK AFTER YOUR HAIR

Washing you hair is not so much for health as for appearance; six times a year would keep it healthy but probably looking awful. So it really depends on how it is worn, and what you see in the mirror. Try washing it every 6 to 10 days. If it is oily you will need to wash more often, if dry, less. But be careful, the stimulation of the washing action itself can spur the oil glands in the follicles to produce yet more sebum making the condition worse. With oily hair always rinse with cool water and don't use a highly alkaline detergent shampoo. Harsh shampoos can strip the oils off your hair completely and encourage the sebaceous glands to produce even more. If your hair is dry, always use a conditioner. There are many things you'll find in the kitchen that can be put to use for hair health and beauty. Try some of these:

To gently brighten and lighten blonde hair:
Boil a cup of dried camomile flowers in a pint of water for 15 minutes. Strain and pour through hair as a final rinse every time you wash.

To add shimmer:
Boil a bunch of fresh parsley in a pint of water for 15 minutes and pour through hair as a final rinse.

To give deep lustre to dark hair:
Steep 3 tablespoons of rosemary in a pint of water for 15 minutes and use as a final rinse.

To restore health to dry, brittle hair:
Beat two eggs together with 2 tbls. each of olive oil and honey 1 tble. of cidar vinegar. Shampoo as usual, rinse then apply all-honey massaging, well into hair and scalp. Cover with a towel, wait for 15 minutes, shampoo and rinse.

DANDRUFF

This annoying problem comes in two forms, dry and scaly, flaking off easily onto shoulders, or thick greasy scales that stick to the scalp. In both cases the cause is unknown. Medicated shampoos can help to get rid of scales and discourage their reappearance; the strongest contain zinc pyrothionate. But they can be very harsh on skin and scalp if used often. Sometimes washing your hair every two or three days in a one per cent solution of cetrimide, an antiseptic detergent, will do the trick.

Brush it daily to remove dust, dirt, waste and dead cells from scalp and to stimulate a good blood supply to the scalp. Always use a good comb, preferably one that is saw cut and made of bone, ivory or vulcanised rubber. Keep combs and brushes immaculate to prevent infection.

Have your hair cut or trimmed regularly. Although cutting will not make hair grow any faster it will make it look thicker and healthier.

Massage can help a head of hair to look better, grow faster, and feel better too. It increases blood flow to the scalp. Place your fingers deep into the hair and move your scalp in a circular motion firmly, leaving the fingers in one place, never sliding them over the surface of the scalp. Then change the position and do the same thing again until the whole scalp area has been covered.

If you bleach, dye or perm your hair, seek professional advice first. Some of the worst damage done to hair is by improper treatment in these areas. 233

Eyes, Ears and Teeth

EYES

Your eyes are highly complex and magnificent organs, capable of transmitting vast quantities of information to the brain in split seconds. But they are also quite delicate instruments, and to preserve their wonderful qualities they need a certain amount of care and attention.

The quality of light around you is important, especially when you are involved in close or finicky work. Good clear north light is the best, but if that's not possible, make sure you buy a good lamp with a bright clear bulb. Put it behind your left shoulder if you are right-handed, so that the light falls on your work. Very often people talk about your eyes being tired, or needing a rest. But the eye is basically a muscle, and if it is healthy, then it isn't your eyes that are tired, it's your brain. Take a break from whatever you are doing, go for a walk, work on something else for a while, or even have a catnap. You'll get up feeling refreshed and ready to begin again. If you are feeling tired, and you have to go out for the evening, lie down with your eyes covered for five or ten minutes. Cotton pads moistened with cool water or witch hazel over your closed lids will help your whole face to feel refreshed, too.

Check your eyes regularly – as we get older, many conditions change. Children particularly may be suffering from some sort of defect which is easily correctable with the right glasses. Contact lenses are a useful aid for men and women who find themselves uncomfortable in ordinary glasses. The new lenses are much more comfortable these days, and they are easier to handle.

When you order glasses, don't forget to ask for sunglasses as well if you think you are going to need them. But don't get in the habit of thinking they are a fashion accessory like a handbag or a necklace. They are very useful when the sun is glaring, on the beach during the height of summer, or when you are surrounded by snow. But walking around 365 days of the year in a brown or blue haze doesn't do you *or* your eyes any good.

TEETH

In theory your teeth should be the easiest parts of your body to keep strong and healthy – they are hard, resistant to damage, protected by the mouth, and most of us have been thoroughly brain-washed by toothpaste ads and dentist's warnings. Yet in reality, teeth get an enormous amount of wear and tear, and they suffer more than the delicate eyes and ears which appear so vulnerable.

To begin with, we eat far too much concentrated sugars and sweeteners which stimulate bacteria to form in the mouth. These in turn combine with tiny particles of food to form a nasty substance called plaque, coating the surface of the teeth. Plaque attracts acids which start to eat their way into the enamel, wearing it away and gradually dissolving it. Without treatment, the bacteria then invade the dentine, or inner part of the tooth, and form a cavity. The pulp may become inflamed and painful, and if it goes unchecked, you may develop an abcess in the root. A sad story, and all too common. Cavities can be discouraged from forming in

234

the first place in two ways; first, eat as little sugar and sugary products as possible, brush your teeth regularly after every meal and use special gum sticks to massage the gums between the teeth to remove any last remaining particles of food, and keep the circulation going so that the teeth remain strongly rooted in the gum, and the gum itself stays healthy.

BRUSHING YOUR TEETH

Use your toothbrush at least twice a day, using a short tough bristle that won't damage or scratch the enamel. Brush repeatedly in one direction only, up and down, on the inside and outside surfaces. Then brush across the tops of the flat molars. Use dental floss or gum massage sticks to remove all particles and throw them away immediately after use. Never use toothpicks with sharp points – they can pierce the delicate gum and cause infection.

EARS

Your ears are a very precious part of your body, and they have suffered comparatively little damage in the past, except for unwise poking and probing.

Today the noise of ordinary life has reached ridiculous proportions, and we all are only too aware of how much the city sounds and traffic noise can affect our need for some peace and at least a few quiet hours. Ears are responsible for more than hearing, though, the inner ear controls our balance too, so that when this gets out of kilter we may find it difficult to walk.

Inside the ear canal that leads from the outside into the inner ear, tiny glands secrete a wax called cerumen. This makes sure that small insects and flies are prevented from getting inside into the ear drum, and it also keeps out particles of dust and dirt which get caught up in the sticky flakes. Sometimes this wax accumulates in larger quantities than normal, and you may be tempted to try and remove it yourself by syringing. Don't. Putting anything into the ear can be dangerous, and especially if children see you and copy it themselves with pencils or a sharp object. Get your doctor to syringe your ears now and then if necessary.

For most people daily ear care is simple – a gentle wash with your usual soap and water. Tipped soft swabs will take away sticky dirt from the outer crevices; never *ever* use a pointed stick instead.

As we get older, the acuteness of our hearing may diminish considerably. This is con sidered a natural part of aging. But it can have a very unnatural effect by isolating you from normal life. Never be ashamed to say you can't hear, and get a hearing aid as soon as you realize that you've begun to keep away from other people because you can't understand them anyway. Modern aids are almost invisible, but any aid is better than a world of silence.

Children often have problems that go unnoticed because they react by simply opting out, or going about their own business without appearing to listen to the teacher. Check your child's hearing regularly.

WHEN NATURE NEEDS A LITTLE HELP

Nobody likes to get old-looking. And although aging cannot be put off for ever, it can be slowed down by using a few simple tricks; daily exercises to tone and firm the muscles of the face, a little massage to boost circulation and iron out lines and wrinkles and a few treatments to keep skin glowing smooth and healthy. And not just for women. Men's skin needs care too, although they are lucky simply because they shave every day. Shaving is one method of exfoliation, that is, scraping off the outer dead layers of the skin. Many dermatologists believe this stimulates the reproduction of skin cells (which slows down with the passing of the years) and keeps a face looking smooth, and glowing. No one would suggest that women shave, but they can get the same gentle abrasive action by using a grainy soap or cleanser once a week for dry skin, two or three times if it is oily. Make your own by mixing together a cup of finely ground steel-cut oatmeal with a cup of sweet almond oil. Just before washing, rub the skin well with the mixture for a couple of minutes, then rinse away the excess. Finally, wash as normal. Regular exfoliation, plus five minutes of face exercises and a minute or two of massage after shaving or before your bath or shower, will bring lasting results.

Take advantage of cosmetics, too, but remember the powdered and painted look is gone. A modern face should look glowing and healthy, individual and above all natural. Get the most from cosmetics by bringing out your best features and giving you a glow of health.

236

THE FABULOUS FIVE FACE SAVERS

To avoid and correct a double chin
Lie on your back on a bed, shoulders and neck supported by the bed with your head just over the edge so it falls backwards. Relax completely. Now slowly raise head, chin first until your chin touches your chest to a count of five. Slowly lower again to the same count until you're back to the completely relaxed position. Repeat five times.

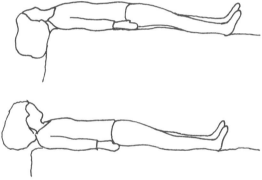

To stimulate circulation and tighten muscles all over the face
Standing in front of a mirror, open your eyes and mouth as far as you can as though you were silently screaming … really pulling all of the muscles in your face tight and taut, to a slow count of five. Now let go, relaxing the whole face slowly. Repeat three times.

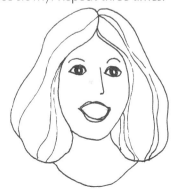

To firm mouth and jaw area
Open your mouth as wide as possible and toss your head back. Now open and close your mouth a dozen times by moving the lower jaw.

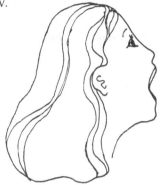

To ease scowl lines
Place the palm of one hand flat and firm against the centre of your forehead covering the area between the eyes. Put your elbow against a firm surface such as a desk or table to give support to the hand. Pressing down with your head against your hand so the skin is held firm, 'scowl', pulling your forehead muscles in hard to a slow count of three. Now to the same slow count of three relax them completely. Repeat five times.

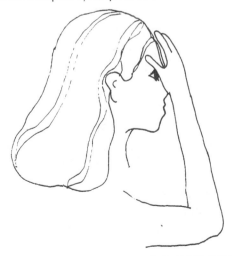

wear a piece of clear tape or adhesive tape over the scowl area when you're at home alone. It will help to iron out lines and make you aware of the unconscious muscle action that put them there in the first place.

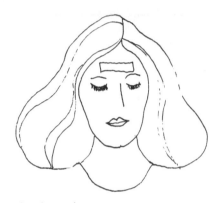

For cheeks and eyes
Placing the palms of your hands firmly against your upper cheeks and temples on either side of your face (elbows sticking out at right angles to the head) press in while you 'smile up' crinkling your eyes and drawing the corners of the mouth and cheeks upward to a count of three. Now relax the position to the same count of three.

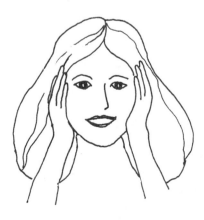

OTHER TREATMENTS:

Cool pick-me-up

This works wonders after a long hard day. It is also the best and cheapest toner for the skin, boosting circulation beautifully. Good for all types of skin except for broken veins. Fill a bowl or basin with cold water, and add a tray of ice-cubes. Dressed warmly, and wearing rubber gloves (so your hands don't freeze) splash the cold water on your face. Begin with six splashes the first time and gradually work up to twenty as your skin gets used to the treatment. Blot dry with a towel and apply a moisturizer.

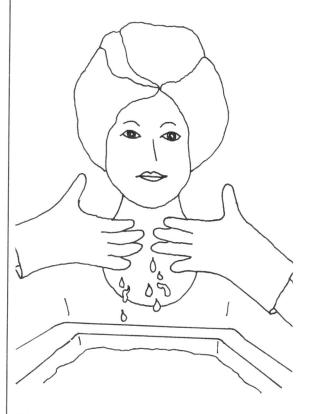

Steam cleaning

Great for oily skin, this treatment clears out clogged pores and really deep cleans. Put a few leaves of mint, camomile, rosemary, or comfrey into a pot of water just off the boil. Put your face above it and cover your head with a towel so your skin gets the steam and stay there for three to five minutes. Cleanse with an exfoliator, splash with cool water, pat dry, and apply a moisturizer.

Forehead smoothing

Face relaxed, lips together, stroke from one side of the forehead to the other alternating hands, so the right fingers of the right hand will start at the left temple and stroke across to the right, followed by the fingers of the left hand starting at the right temple and ending at the left one. Repeat with each hand six times then, using both at the same time, stroke upwards from the brows to the hairline six times.

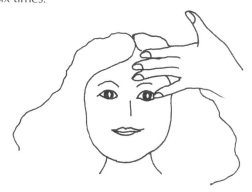

Face massage is gentler and lighter than body massage and is done using the second, third and fourth fingers of the hand together. You can do it for five or ten minutes watching television or in the bath, smoothing out tension, softening lines and improving the circulation.

Throat and chin strokes

With your mouth closed and chin raised run fingers up from the chest over the neck and under the chin in long smooth strokes coming off at the chin. Start at the outsides of the neck and move further in with each stroke. Repeat a dozen times.

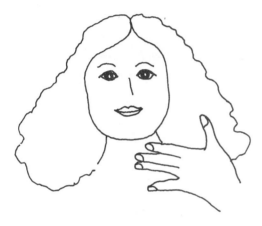

Mouth and chin strokes

Bring the lips together in a firm and hard 'O' shape as if you are saying 'woo'. Now stroke with fingers up from chin and mouth area outwards over cheeks and ending at the ears. Repeat a dozen times.

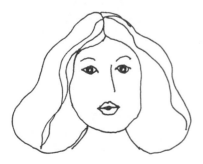

Mouth and temple strokes

With your mouth in the same pursed shape, stroke upwards and outwards over top of cheeks and out to temples. Repeat a dozen times.

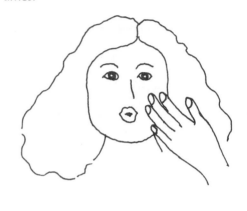

FOR MEN, TOO

Men are funny about their faces. They worry about lines and sags but seldom bother to do anything to prevent either. The skin on a man's face ages slowly or rapidly in direct proportion to the care he takes of it. And, constantly exposed to sun, wind and weather – not to mention the products of air pollution – it does need care. It needs protection from the ultra-violet rays of the sun which age the skin rapidly. A good sun-screen will do, but choose one that offers high protection, or use a moisturizer with a sun-screen in it. Put it on after shaving in the morning and again in the middle of the day, if you wash you face. Alcohol-based aftershaves can be very drying – you are better with a lotion after-shave, or use a good moisturizer after applying an alcohol-based one.

239

HANDS

Hands are one of the most expressive parts of your body. They reveal your age, tell much about how you live, and display your character and personality in the way you use them. Often treated roughly, hands are also the most neglected part of the body.

In all there are 28 bones that make your hand and wrist, arranged to give the maximum flexibility. They are amazing tools. Extremely tough yet highly sensitive. They re-act badly to harsh weather (particularly extremes of heat or cold) prolonged exposure to the sun which tends to turn them blotchy and produce so-called liver spots. These blemishes which increase with age, have nothing to do with the liver are the result of a high concentration of pigment in clusters because of the skin re-action to the ultra-violet rays of the sun. Once your hands have become really neglected it is difficult to 'rejuvenate' and revitalize them completely. By far the best

method of looking after hands is a simple routine of day-to-day prevention.

HOW TO LOOK AFTER YOUR HANDS

1. Keep them away from harsh chemicals, detergents, and cleansers by wearing rubber gloves for wet jobs in the house and cotton or leather gloves in the garden. (The cotton-lined type of rubber glove is most comfortable).
2. Protect hands from wind and weather with gloves in the winter and a good strong sunscreen cream in the summer.
3. Every time you wet or wash your hands, pat them dry, then apply a good hand cream or lotion containing silicon which acts as protection for the skin.
4. Treat rough skin and cracks by bleaching stains with lemon juice and then removing the rough skin with a pumice stone. Finish off by rubbing in a rich hand cream or simple vegetable oil. (This treatment has to be repeated several times to see results in bad cases.)
5. Never wash hands more than absolutely necessary. Every time you use soap it removes the oils from the backs of the hands that are necessary to keep them soft and pliable. Rinsing hands in a mild vinegar and water solution after washing helps protect them from chapping.

NAILS

Nails are mostly keratin and consist of a plate of horny cells which extend beyond the finger tips, plus another part known as the matrix or nail bed, just as long, which remains hidden underneath the cuticles and extends back

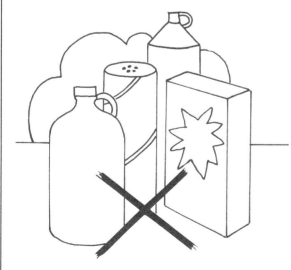

into the finger up to the first joint. The part of the nail we see is dead. The other, invisible part is alive, fed by the blood stream and exists totally to produce the dead part. When any damage is done to your nail, or it falls off because of injury or infection, the damage is completely repairable, for so long as the matrix behind the cuticle remains intact it continues to produce new and perfect nails. To some extent the condition of your nails and their strength depends on inheritance. But nutrition plays a big role too. Nails, like hair, need protein, and indeed like the rest of your body vitamins and minerals particularly. When you are ill your nails suffer. They can become brittle and split easily, weak and flaky, or heavily lined with horizontal ridges. With improved nutrition and good day-to-day care these problems will soon grow out and disappear. Vertical ridges tend to appear with age and are particularly common in people suffering from rheumatism. They can also indicate excessive dryness.

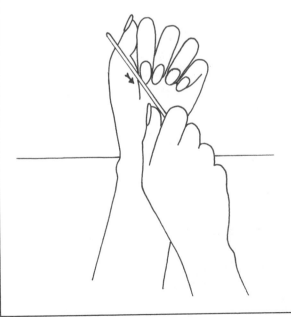

White spots that appear from time to time on nails can be the result of injury, a zinc deficiency, over-acidity of the system, or stress. They grow out and disappear as the nail grows … at the rate of about $\frac{1}{4}$ inch a month. The more you use your hands particularly the tips of your fingers, for instance, in playing the piano or typewriting the faster nails will grow.

HOW TO LOOK AFTER YOUR NAILS

Remember that your nails can be damaged easily and it takes time for the damage to grow out so special care is needed to prevent trouble in the first place.

1. Keep nails shaped by filing in an oval from each side of the nail to the centre only. Never use a metal file – they tend to split the nail. Emery boards are better.
2. Try not to cut cuticles. It can lead to infection of the matrix and possible long-term nail problems. Instead keep them soft by the daily application of a rich hand or cuticle cream to that dry patches and splits don't appear in the first place. If you must remove a cuticle do it carefully, applying an antiseptic afterwards and cutting from around the nail only.
3. If nails are weak, take powdered gelatin daily dissolved in fruit juice – a spoonful should be enough. Apply white iodine to them daily or one of the nail hardeners you can buy in a chemist. Clear nail varnish can help too to strengthen them and keep them from splitting. Improve overall nutrition.

FATIGUE

Women are more prone to chronic fatigue than men. Partly this is because in her day-to-day life caring for a family a woman is far less likely to pay heed to the signals that she needs rest and do something about it. She will usually put her husband and her children's needs before her own until fatigue becomes compounded and turns into a chronic problem. Fatigue can have a nutritional basis too. Mothers at home with young children neglect nutrition because they can't be bothered to prepare anything for themselves.

Low blood sugar can also be a cause. So can anaemia. Because of the blood loss through menstruation many women find it difficult to maintain a high enough level of red blood cells. But anaemia is not something that should be self-diagnosed and then treated with a course of iron pills or a tonic. There are many possible causes which need to be investigated before the proper treatment can be given. If you suspect anaemia, go to your doctor and let him give you a blood test to find out. Then he will prescribe treatment.

Some women appear to have a very high requirement for the B-complex vitamins. No one is sure why this is so. There seems to be a link between the level of oestrogen a woman produces and her need for these vitamins.

Adding a B-complex supplement that contains the full range of these vitamins in a good balance, can often go a long way towards changing things. So can exercise. Just because you are on your feet all day

doesn't mean you are getting enough exercise. Regular exercise, say, swimming or running three times a week can help a lot to banish tiredness.

Much fatigue is mental in origin. It can come from boredom with a life that doesn't offer enough mental stimulation. Perhaps there is a hobby or interest you could take up to get you out of your rut. Should you be taking on a new challenge? Are you stretching yourself enough? These are some of the important things to consider when you find yourself suffering from a feeling of tiredness that doesn't seem to want to go away.

LEG ACHES AND VARICOSE VEINS

Swollen veins occur when the tissues of blood vessels become weakened yet still have to deal with the hard work of carrying blood back to the heart.

Tiny valves that open and close alternatively keep the blood flowing in the right direction towards the heart between pulse beats. But if a tissue is weakened, a valve may not close completely, then there is a back-flow of blood on to the valve below. This adds weight to the lower valve and increases the volume and pressure within the vein. The wall of the vein stretches and as a result, you develop a varicose.

The best way to avoid varicose veins is to see that you are not overweight and don't allow yourself to suffer from constipation. Eat as little sugar and flour as possible and get plenty of natural roughage plus bran if necessary. Once they appear, to lessen their discomfort avoid long hours of standing and sitting. When you have been on your feet for some time, relieve the pressure by resting with your legs propped up high. If your work forces you to sit for long periods, make sure you get plenty of exercise – swimming, walking, cycling, dancing, for instance. This will help keep the blood from settling in the lower limbs.

In severe cases you should consult your doctor, but when the condition is mild it can be greatly helped by support hose.

One important point; varicose veins are often due to genetics – mother and daughter will have them in the same leg, even in the same place. If there is a tendency in your family, you have to take extra care especially when you are pregnant. Make sure you don't get overweight, and wear support stockings all the time.

PILL PROBLEMS

Women, just because of their femininity, experience a group of health problems that are hormone related. Almost every woman during her fertile life is aware of the floodtides and the ebbs of her hormones. To most women it is just this – an awareness. To others, however, it is much more than this and a problem called premenstrual tension has to be solved. Good news is that today it can be solved although there is no universal solution, no magic pill that suits everybody.

Doctors solve the problem of premenstrual tension by treating the symptoms the victim finds most upsetting. If this is fluid retention a diuretic pill will encourage the body's usually excellent fluid balance system to get back into gear. If mood changes are the main worry and a usually pleasant woman finds herself turning for several days each month into a crabby old creature who hates herself and everyone else, hormone supplements often bring her back to normal good health. At times if depression is uppermost in the premenstrual syndrome an antidepressive drug or a pyridoxine (Vitamin B6) supplement eliminates a life of intermittent misery.

A good example of how complex and individual the female response is to her hormones is demonstrated by a miserable side effect of the (contraceptive) Pill. The commonest reason for women coming off the pill as their chosen contraceptive is a type of depressive illness in which the joy of life seems to ebb away and sexual interest wanes and disappears. Quite recently doctors have found this is linked once again with Vitamin B6 deficiency.

But strangely this deficiency appears in only half of the cases of Pill depression. In these cases, in which the Pill induces a very low or even an absence of pyridoxine in the blood, the mood changes can be reversed by giving a daily supplement of the vitamin. This can be given in a sustained release form which gently supplements the victim back to health and vigour. Those women who are not pyridoxine deficient and get depressed on the Pill only have one other option – to change to a different form of contraception.

THE CHANGE OF LIFE

No change at all is what happens to at least ten per cent of all women when they get to the menopause. Another ten per cent need some sensible medication to get them through a troublesome time. The rest do experience a change. But it's not anywhere near as bad as they expected and this raises a highly interesting point. Why is the change, the menopause, the climacteric – call it what you like – such a worry point in so many women's lives.

I think the answer lies in history. Doctoring by and large was pretty terrible within our composite folk knowledge and that is for present generations the 19th Century. And if doctors in general were not very clever and sending for the doctor was, generally speaking, pretty near to sending for the undertaker, doctoring for what were euphemistically called 'female complaints' was really dreadful. Gynaecology was the last full blown speciality to develop within the general fabric of medicine and before gynaecologists developed their own expertise some pretty nasty things were done to women. And as for their 'female complaints' these were either put down to their inherent frigidity or their ravenous nymphomania. So naturally they tended to look elsewhere for help and help came mostly from empirics and quacks.

Both of these professions were in an ideal situation to get a wide following – for they could do at least one thing that other doctors couldn't do and remain in practice. They could advertise and advertise they did. One of the pioneers in this field was Mrs. Lydia Pinkum from Lynne, Massachusetts who had an enormously successful following with a folk medicine remedy she found in an old pharmacopoeia. She finished up as the first lady of the successful handling of the menopause and also the first lady millionaire it is said.

Of course she had many less well known colleagues. Often they exploited the symptoms of the menopause and built up the enormous cultural hangover of fear and dread that hangs over this rather interesting and exclusively human physical change in the life of all women.

Of course we all change in scores of ways as the years go by. The physiology of the body alters and it's not realistic to sit down and add up all the bad things about aging and forget the advantages. You may feel you would like to look 18 years old. But how many of us would really like to be a teenager again? Or a young mother with a new baby to manage? Or to be struggling to climb those early corner steps once more?

The changes of the change of life are well documented. Most of them when they are really troublesome are due to a sudden turn off of the ovary's oestrogen production. You don't lose it all for the body makes some in other glands that go on functioning until the day you die. But it's not quite as easy as that. Daily ovarian oestrogen production has a regular system in the pituitary gland that also regulates all sorts of automatic body functions – fluid balance for instance. In a way it is a bit like an oven thermostat – it's unthinkingly automatic. When oestrogen levels fall the pituitary whips itself up to signal more. But the ovaries are shutting up the shop and can't oblige, so the pituitary really starts sending out its automatic distress symptom demands. These can't do a lot as far as oestrogen is concerned (but it does do something on that score). It does, however, have one great success (in its unthinking automatic reaction) it stirs up a whole lot of other systems too. And these produce the symptoms associated with the change of life.

Keeping fit is about keeping normal, doing your own thing and living your life and enjoying it. If the menopause interferes with this do something about it. It doesn't *have* to be hormone replacement therapy although that helps sometimes. All sorts of tailor made treatments help with the very diverse symptoms that worry some women at this time. But don't expect to be ill. Don't expect to say goodbye to being a woman, or goodbye to being sexual. Margaret Mead has studied the sexuality of women in almost every culture and is on record as saying that female sexuality persists for as long as it is *expected* to exist in every culture.

This must not be taken as saying that you don't get sexual symptoms at the menopause. Many symptoms are experienced more commonly at one age than another from babyhood onwards. But today you can usually do something about worrying symptoms. See a good doctor.

BREAST CHECK

It is a good idea to examine your breasts every couple of months. Most breast cancer is controllable provided it is diagnosed early enough, and the best preliminary check possible is one you can do on your own. Here's how:
Standing undressed to the waist in front of a mirror, with arms at your sides, look for any irregularities in the outline of your breasts or any dimpling or puckering of the skin. Then look at the nipples to be sure there has been no discharge or bleeding.

Now lie down with a pillow under your head and your right arm behind your head. With your left hand, fingers flat, run your hand in a circular motion around the right breast moving closer to the centre with each circle. Examine the armpits too, looking for any new lumps or tender spots. Now change hands and examine the left breast. If you find anything unusual make an appointment with your doctor at once. *Most lumps and irritations are not serious problems,* but your doctor should check them as soon as you find something. If a lump needs medical attention, the quicker it is treated, the better. If it is nothing, your mind will be at ease.

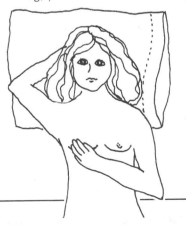

Especially For Men

A POT BELLY

One of the most unattractive features any man can have is a pot belly. It makes him look older, sloppy, and can even lead to long-term back trouble because of excess strain the extra flesh puts on back muscles. Besides, there is little excuse when it is such an easy thing to get rid of. If you are over-weight, see our section on diet and get rid of the excess pounds, beginning an exercise program at the same time. If not, all you need is the exercise, although it does matter *what* you eat! The most common nutritional cause of a pot belly is taking in too many refined carbohydrates … white bread and stuff made from white flour, sugary things and especially too much beer. Jogging or running is particularly good for trimming the middle. Here are two special abdominal exercises to do, if possible, several times a day for quick results:

Isometric abdominal hold:
Standing straight, pull in your abdominal muscles as hard as you can. It should feel as though your stomach is pressing against your backbone. During the contraction breathe normally and see that the tension is taken in your middle only, not in your shoulders, limbs or head. Hold for six seconds then release. Repeat six times. As you get used to the exercise you can extend the periods of contraction until you are holding your stomach in for a full minute, twice in succession with a few seconds in-between. Repeat this three times a day.

THINNING HAIR

One in five men in the West will go at least partially bald. And, sad to tell, if you happen to be the one there is not a great deal you can do about it. Hair loss is largely hereditary. There are innumerable, supposedly 'sure fire' treatments for hair loss that are supposed to restore growth.

However, there are ways of holding back – and in some cases even stopping – hair loss if you catch it soon enough.

First, keep your hair clean by using a mild pH balanced shampoo as often as necessary. This will help stop excessive dryness, oiliness and scaling. Then protect your hair from the sun, chemicals such as harsh shampoos, chlorine in swimming pools, and heavy brushing or too vigorous massage which could harm it. Be sure you keep really fit physically through good nutrition One of the most common causes of hair loss is excess tension and worry. Finally, have your hair looked at periodically by a dermatologist or a qualified tricologist, and don't be taken in by unscrupulous sellers of dreams.

If you do lose your hair, by far the best thing is to come to terms with it instead of trying to hide it. Have it cut well and don't ever let it seem that you are trying to cover up a balding patch by combing a few wisps of hair over a shiny head. It looks terrible. If you hair loss has been widespread, you might even consider shaving your head. It can look great.

MALE MENOPAUSE

There is much controversy about whether or not men undergo a change comparable to the menopause in women. From a hormonal point of view some studies show a decline in the production of testosterone after 45 or 50, while other studies of men of all ages between 20 and 93 indicate that levels are about the same in all age groups. Nevertheless, many men after the age of forty-five experience a decline in sexual capacity. But there are so many things that can be responsible for that.

Probably the most common symptom associated with so-called male menopause is chronic fatigue and muscular weakness. On a psychological level there are also reports of irritability, insomnia and anxiety. For many reasons this period of middle life can be very difficult.

Men in this age group tend to be physically less fit, not because they are older but because most of them have neglected themselves, particularly if they are involved in office work. Lack of exercise, too much of the wrong kind of foods, coffee, alcohol and stimulants, plus cigarettes, and the pressures from job problems and business achievements (or the lack of them) all take their toll. Often men at this age experience a feeling of no longer being needed and a sense of confusion about life goals. It is a time for re-assessment, for leaving behind the old and finding a new sense of values to face the future with. All of these things can affect a man's feelings of virility and his interest and performance in sex.

Trimming away excess pounds and slowly easing yourself into a demanding and regular exercise routine will usually improve your sexual drive and performance greatly. It will also help you deal with excessive anxiety and give you some time to yourself and the space you may need to re-assess where you are going and what is important to you now. This is also a time when enormous courage and honesty is needed between men and women about sex, about themselves and each other, and about what they want and don't want from their future lives.

But feelings of worry, fatigue and discouragement, far from being signs that you are losing your youth and therefore your manhood, are far more likely to be an indication that change is coming, and you simply need to adjust yourself to a different attitude towards yourself and your life.

This can be the beginning of the most satisfying and fulfilling period of your life. Tenderness and skill can make sex into something far more satisfying than anything you have ever known – you have a lifetime of experience to pour into a relationship that can only grow in closeness and pleasure, and practically speaking, you have more time, too. Use it positively and creatively. For perhaps the first time since you were a child, take the time to think about yourself, something young men on their way up forget about. There will never be a better time, if you have the good sense to understand.

Sleep: Fact and Fiction

HOW MUCH DO YOU NEED TO SLEEP?

Few people realize it, but regular and sufficient sleep is the best way to look your best. When you are rested, your eyes are clear and alert, your skin is toned up and radiant, your overall appearance is vigorous and full of life. Your brain works at its top level, too, and your whole expression is relaxed and unworried.

Most of us have a lot of funny notions about sleep. The idea that everyone needs that magic eight hours is simply untrue. Sleep needs vary from one person to another, and change during various periods of life. Sometimes you may require as little as four hours a night, at others as much as eleven – there are no hard and fast rules.

Sleeping is a way of restoring energy, relieving stress and worry, and even speeding up healing processes in the body. And, in spite of all our medical knowledge, there is still something mysterious, almost magical, about this state which is so necessary to us that we spend a third of our lives in it.

Basically there are two sleep patterns. The first is called orthodox sleep when the blood pressure, breathing rate and brain-wave activities are all lowered. Most of each night is spent in this state, which is primarily the great physical restorer. Our brainwaves become calm and synchronized and all our body's systems tick over at a slow ebb. But the production of antibodies to fight infection and the speed at which our cells are restored both greatly increase. We also let go of all the tensions that result in achy shoulders and sore backs.

The second kind of sleep is called paradoxical sleep because in many ways it seems to be a mass of contradictions. Brainwaves are very active, breathing speeds up and we make involuntary physical movements. Paradoxical sleep is also known as REM because of rapid eye movements beneath the closed lids that show the sleeper is dreaming.

What orthodox sleep does for the body, REM sleep and dreaming seem to do for the mind. It appears to be vital for our mental and emotional health, to help us resolve difficulties, conflicts and mental pressures. Although they are very different from each other, both orthodox and REM sleep are essential to mental and physical health. We sleep in well defined patterns every night alternating between the two, ninety minutes of orthodox sleep separated by ten to twenty minute periods of REM.

If you were awakened every time the REM stage began you would suffer from increased anxiety, worries, poor concentration and depression during your waking hours. Deprived of REM for a week or two, you'd show every sign of 'REM rebound'. This means that every night there would be REM periods than usual, often with nightmares or frightening dreams, or sometimes even hallucinations. When mind and body are satisfied that they've made up for the loss, sleep patterns will return to normal.

One of the dangers of taking sleeping pills for longer than a few days is that they can repress REM, and lead to temporary but frightening REM rebound when they are given up. There are other reasons to avoid using drugs for sleeplessness. Taken regularly, they gradually lose their effectiveness as the body demands more to put you to sleep. Many barbituates can also become seriously addictive.

Of course, when real difficulties occur in your life like serious illness, loss of a job, or money problems, it is not surprising that you may spend a few sleepless nights tossing and turning. You would have to be superhuman to avoid worrying. But if you maintain general good health you should be able to cope without doing your mind or body any great harm. During times like these it is even more important to get enough exercise, and eat well.

Ordinarily, how much sleep you need depends entirely on you. Some geniuses and high achievers such as Napoleon, Thomas Edison, and Freud slept very little. Others, like Einstein, could sleep the day away. One thing is sure: the less you worry about going to sleep, the less likely you are to have trouble doing it.

HOW TO GET TO SLEEP

Drugs are not the answer except for occasional times of great stress, and only with your doctor's advice. Getting to sleep is more often a question of what you don't do, instead of what you do.

● Don't exercise just before bedtime. It is far too stimulating to your whole system. But do exercise during the day to relieve tension and muscle strain.

● Don't drink coffee or other stimulating beverages at dinner, and try a glass of milk or cocoa just before getting into bed.

● Don't go to bed when you're not sleepy. Read a light novel, listen to quiet music, sew, or just sit and relax.

● Don't sleep during the day, even if you are tired. Practice a relaxation technique instead for ten minutes during the afternoon, and just before dinner.

● Get to know the natural tranquillizers which have been used by herbalists for centuries, and take a cup half an hour before bedtime. Try camomile, skullcap, catnip, or passion-flower teas, which you can buy in tablet form in many health stores.

● Take a lukewarm (not hot) bath, and submerge for ten minutes at least. Dry off slowly, then quickly get into bed.

● Get into a routine so you go to bed at the same time every night, and perform the same ritual (cat out, teeth brushed, etc.). The mind loves patterns, and learns to expect to go to sleep.

● When you can't sleep, don't worry about it. Put the light on and read, write, or just let your mind wander. If you don't sleep tonight, you will tomorrow, or the next night.

Mind and Body Together

Introduction

THE FINAL SCORE

In the beginning is the child, born with a whole set of programmed characteristics as a result of that fabulously dangerous but exciting game of chromosome dice we all play when we make a baby. A combination of inherited genes may turn out a mathematical genius or jazz-loving saxophone player, or both in the same human being. Perhaps the throw of the dice will bring a tendency towards heart disease, or the constitution of an ox with a temperament to match; a shape like an all-in wrestler or the delicate bone structure of a wistful elf.

But that is truly only the beginning. From birth onwards, all these characteristics can be modified and adapted, giving the best possible chance for good health in every aspect of life. For most of this book, we have concentrated on the physical aspects of good health, the body and its function of keeping you fit and well for as long as you live. We have spoken about good nutrition and healthy, pleasurable eating; we've seen how supple and mobile bodies keep us in trim, our hearts, lungs and muscles working together to make a strong sturdy foundation for useful living and enjoyment; and finally, we've shown how to take good care of your newly delightful body so that you look as good as you feel.

But just as it's become popular to say 'it's not all in the mind', perhaps it's time to stop and realize that it's not all in the body either. We are truly remarkable creatures, and our thoughts and dreams are as tangible a part of our bodies as fingers and toes. The smallest baby becomes physically ill when the world is a hostile place, and blossoms into smiling chuckling contentment when the world is full of love and affection.

The lack of warmth and openly-expressed love is one of the greatest problems in this frantic complicated century. Love is a good health factor more potent than sunshine or penicillin. It's a natural food of life which ought to be on every shelf and in every home.

We know that we need each other, we understand that babies need tender loving care, and older children need cuddling and affection more than they need good food. But stresses and strains get in the way; we are distracted by anxieties and worries which seem temporarily more important. We promise ourselves that when a few quiet moments come, we'll stop and listen, we'll stop and learn to love again.

The years slide by as we scrape and save to give our families financial security, a better house, a nicer car, a new suit. The children grow up, they seem to be more independent anyway, and we turn away again preoccupied with their physical well-being, until suddenly it's too late. We've forgotten how to say 'I love you'.

Well, it needn't be like that. There is a better way to live, a healthier way, and if you have come this far, then you should know by now that it is truly never too late. It's not too late to re-organize your life along with your shape.

Not too late for dieting, or getting fit or changing the way you look, and especially not too late for love. Good health and good loving go along together, part of you from the inside out. It is being able to reach inside yourself for that unexpected strength and calm whenever you need it most. It is understanding that *Mind and Body together* is the summing up of everything we've talked about in the book, and especially your attitude to yourself, to your family, and to everyone around you.

It is being able to take a deep breath before you explode – you may explode anyway, but that one moment of respite will let you see a little more clearly, and you'll be able to deal with the problem afterwards in a more constructive way.

Of course love and quiet contentment won't solve all your difficulties. It won't get you a new job or pay the rent, or cure a broken leg, although it will help you work things out. And there are times when we think it is worth the sacrifice to gain some security or a package deal we think we can make up when things are better.

Well, perhaps it was worth it. Everyone must decide for themselves, as long as the decision is taken with open eyes.

Be warned. Your state of mind, your feelings and your dreams matter. You can't help anyone else until you are in the best of health through and through, and *pay now fly later* can all too easily become *pay now and die sooner.* Not such a good deal for your family, either, so take a very good look …

You & Your Self-image

THE MIRROR SELF

When you look in the mirror, what do you see? One of the most extraordinary things about all human beings is that almost always we see someone quite different from the person our friends and family know. If you have a positive picture of yourself, if you truly *like* the person that you are, then you will automatically see someone pleasant, friendly, and interesting – someone you would like to know. But if you think of yourself as weak, ugly, stupid or worthless, then that is exactly what you'll see in the mirror. Each time you look at yourself, that negative feeling will be reinforced by the sight of someone you don't like, someone uninteresting, miserable and unpleasant.

But mirrors aren't magic, except in fairy tales, and the different reflections are objectively the same person. Your hair and eyes, your face and your body don't really change; the mirror that turns you from what you are, to what you *think* you are, is a creation of your own brain, and the person you see is a picture of what you think.

It's an interesting example of the power of the mind, but is it that important? Do we really need to see clearly, so that we can change what we can, and learn to accept what we cannot change? The answer from every viewpoint is an emphatic, overwhelming yes.

To begin with, the very foundation of a warm contented life is a feeling of being comfortable with oneself. Not blindly vain or self-satisfied, just comfortable.

Knowing and appreciating what you are is the greatest strength any human being can possess. With a solid core of generous confidence and understanding, we can reach out easily to other human beings, giving and receiving love, enjoying what is possible, accepting some limitations, yet knowing with quiet certainty that almost anything is possible if you want it enough, enough to be willing to make it happen. Self-knowledge and self-confidence can be the quiet heart of a whirlwind, holding us together against the worst blows of fortune.

Without that strength, we are all diminished, frightened by the unknown, unable to cope with the simplest problems, despising ourselves, and therefore despising other people who love us. After all, they must be blind or foolish to care for anyone so unworthy of affection. An empty core protected by a prickly and defensive cover drives away the very love we need so much.

A better picture of ourselves can help to change that, and renewed confidence spills over into every part of our daily life, the silly and unimportant happenings as well as the major crises which can destroy everything.

When you are happy with yourself, knowing that you are doing your best even in difficult circumstances, then somehow it becomes much easier to actually *do* your best. Even if you've been tired and overworked, worn out with answering perpetual questions and settling quarrels between two demanding children, then sending them both off to bed with a slap won't happen too often. When it does, you won't feel guilty for weeks afterwards, trying to buy back their affection with extra treats or indulgences.

When you are asked to do something you would prefer to avoid, then it's easier to say no pleasantly but firmly, instead of resenting the request, but giving in so that you will be liked and 'respected'. If you lose a parent or someone close to you, then you can grieve freely and openly, without feeling somehow deserted and deprived, as if fate had picked you out as a punishment.

And if your marriage is unhappy, and finally ends, you can face up to that too. Bitterness, anger and guilt are going to be there, but not in such large amounts that you can't begin to find a way back to normal living. It isn't that you will never be angry, never feel guilty or upset! On the contrary. It means accepting that when things become too much for you the first person to forgive is yourself, and then you can move on to better moods and happier times, instead of continuing to wallow in recriminations and martyred anxiety.

So if you've decided that you do want to change an unhappy picture of yourself, how do you go about it? How did it get there in the first place? Most of the picture was painted in childhood, when we first became aware of critical ideas and comments made by parents, teachers and friends. A very young child is totally selfish, and totally self-confident; the whole world seems to revolve around its need for food, warmth and love which is quickly supplied. Then quite suddenly, perceptions change, the world moves back and becomes larger and perhaps a little frightening. The young ego is not so important, instructed about what it should or should not do, taken to school whether it wants to go or not, told to eat this or not eat that – it's quite a shock to realize how small you are, and how large everyone else is.

Most of us adjust quite well, as we hold on to warmth and stability in the family and try our feet in the new world. Exploring is important to all human beings, and with a firm foundation of knowing we are loved and cared for, we can move off with returning self-confidence.

But some of us never recover our balance, or lose it again during the sensitive time of adolescence. A sense of fear and inadequacy can make us ashamed of practically anything – ashamed because we are too fat, or too thin, because we are stupid, or because we are too intelligent, ashamed because we didn't know what to say, or because we said the wrong thing. Then the mirror begins to reflect what you feel. You look and think *fat, unlovable, stupid*, and there, before your very eyes, is fat, unlovable you. Soon the body reflects what you see; if you *know* you are fat already, why bother to watch what you eat? If you *know* you are really unlovable, then you might as well be as nasty and mean as you can, and when you *know* you are stupid, as anyone can see when they look at you, then why bother to study or do your homework?

The same self-deception, taken to extremes is found in many anorexic girls who think they are grossly overweight even when they are starving to death.

So the unhappy cycle begins, and unless you try to break the chain reaction, you will go on seeing a person who didn't exist except in your mind, but who influenced everything you did, eventually you have become what you despise.

Of course there are many ways of changing the image you have, and some people will need professional help to be able to get through the false picture to the reality.

But many of us can learn to appreciate ourselves a little more without such drastic measures. The first steps are simple, and involve getting to know yourself a little better than you do now.

Buy a notebook or a diary, and use it just for putting down your feelings and emotions every day. It's not for dates and appointments, it's for reminding yourself you were happy about the dinner party you cooked for, unhappy about a quarrel with your son, dreaming about what you would have liked to do that day, or what you are looking forward to next year. No one will ever see it, so make it as accurate as you can, and as full of nonsense as you choose. It will seem like a silly thing to do, and maybe even like the heart-throb diary you kept in your teens, but keep writing, and don't re-read the entries for a month.

Then sit down by yourself and read it through as objectively as you can. A pattern should begin to emerge – perhaps you never realized how often you think about getting a job, or giving up work. Or how much you care about wanting to paint, or play the piano, or how desperately you are hoping that your daughter will do some of the things you wanted to do yourself.

If you think often about your own parents, maybe you feel guilty about not having expressed your love enough while they were alive. Resentment at being unattractive may be something you thought you'd grown out of long ago, but there it is, along with a delight in growing plants that you never thought to share with anyone. These are just some of the possibilities of self-discovery.

Not all of it will be pleasant, but it will be what you are, and that is the best beginning. Face to face is much more positive than running away, and when you start to understand what you are and what you want, then you can make your understanding work for you, instead of bottling it all up inside.

You can see that you really do want to change your job, so start to look for re-training schemes, or answer want ads in the newspapers for more suitable places. If you are really unhappy about your children's future, then it's time to see the teacher at school, or ask to see a guidance advisor. If being overweight looms large on the horizon, then you can finally realize it is very important to you, and you'll have a much better chance of sticking to a diet. Classes in make-up and fashion are available once you know that you care about how you look, even if everyone says they love you as you are. If *you* don't like yourself, then do something! If you seem to get upset and worried about unimportant things all the time, then sit down

with yourself, and try to sort out what is
behind your feelings. Perhaps it's as simple as
a physical problem – and it would be best to
have a checkup and a chat with your doctor.

Whatever you find out, you'll also realize that
you are a normal human being, with many
good points you didn't even realize were
there. If you have been honest about writing
it all down, almost certainly you'll find that
you have a deep wish to love and be loved,
to care and be cared for, and expressing
those feelings as openly as possible to those
who love you can be the start of the most
satisfying period of your life. Finally, and it
may take many months and many
notebooks, you should be able to look in the
mirror, and say hello to yourself with a smile.

LIVING TOGETHER, OLD AND NEW WAYS

Living together in a family can be one of the most challenging periods in anyone's life. A varied group of people, of different ages and different temperaments, often with conflicting needs and conflicting ideas – it's a wonder that so many of us manage so well.

But it isn't really surprising that the trend in recent years has been away from the old-fashioned ideal of at least three or four generations, all living together in a single household. We are appalled by the lack of privacy our grandparents suffered, by the over-crowded rooms and relationships that seem tangled up with unhealthy attitudes and complicated kinships, with little or no individual attention.

Today it is very different. The parents almost always live alone with their young children, grandparents may be far away in another town or even another country, older children move to their own homes almost as soon as thay can support themselves. The result is that our problems in living together are diametrically different, too much dependance on one single person, the loneliness of isolation for young mothers and elderly parents, and the overwhelming attention that smothers one or two children, or on a childless husband or wife.

It might be a good idea to have another look at those large and lively families of the past, and see if some of their advantages can be adapted to our own more separated lives.

One of the great benefits was the freedom of choice. When only three or four people are together, they become very dependent on each other for continual love and companionship, and a passing row or unimportant burst of anger can assume terrifying proportions. With a dozen children to choose from, finding a sympathetic friend for a youngster was much easier, and an older cousin or uncle temporarily took the place of an absent or preoccupied parent.

We must learn to extend the household by making sure our children have friends who are welcome to visit, by trying to keep in touch with distant members of the family, talking about them and recollecting stories, and chatting about work and neighbors so there is a real world beyond the front door.

Many children enjoy adult company too, particularly when they are older, and our own friends should be encouraged to feel at home with everyone. All too often, it's the parent who resents the affection a child gives to another adult, but this is a vital part of growing up, and takes some of the pressure off the emotional atmosphere at home, especially when there are problems between children and parents.

Another benefit was the sharing of responsibilities. Even when the oldest male was regarded as the mainstay and chief breadwinner, there were so many people contributing money and services to the one household that the loss of a job could be cushioned, and temporary financial crises could be weathered without too much difficulty. When illness struck, there were other hands to nurse the sick, and take over for a time or forever, if it became necessary. This is harder to cope with in today's way of life; friends and neighbors will help when they can, but the major responsibility does rest squarely on one or two people. It can be eased a little, though, with care and planning. *Both* parents should take the trouble to find out exactly what would happen if the breadwinner was out of work, or fell seriously ill. Both parents should know where all the necessary records are, who to go to in an emergency, and what kind of help would be available from Government departments. As children get older, they should become members of the family who give as well as take, fulfilling their own responsibilities as a matter of course. Even setting the table every night can be a youngster's contribution, and helping around the house should be the natural thing to do, not a case for nagging or bribing with extra pocket money.

When there are fewer members in a household, then all must share, and giving everything without expecting any contribution in return is a poor education for life.

Parents are human beings, not just bottomless cornucopias pouring out food, shelter money and presents.

A practical possibility is remembering that older people whose working lives are almost finished may find a new interest and enjoyment in helping with young children and sharing in responsibilities. Grandparents *and* older aunts and uncles should not be strangers to see once or twice a year on dutiful visits, but a part of ordinary life. It isn't just doing things for them, it's letting them do what they can for you. Baby-sitting once a week while Mother goes to her dancing class, cooking dinner one evening while both parents go out to the movies or visit friends, teaching a budding dressmaker how to turn up a hem, or a young carpenter how to make shelves for the kitchen — whatever they have to offer should be gratefully received and actively encouraged.

Doing too much for someone is sometimes worse than doing nothing — we all need to give as well as take. Knowing that they are welcome will make it easier to ask them to let you alone while you are cooking or gardening, or to keep quiet when you are dealing with tantrums or disobedience in your own way.

The smaller the family unit, the greater the pressure on everybody, and the more everyone needs an escape hatch to be themselves. We all need a strong family tie, to give us strength and courage, but we need a chance to be alone and work out things for ourselves, too. Freedom to talk openly about problems and worries, but freedom to keep some things inside. A balance between the overwhelming closeness of the Victorian household, and the isolation and loneliness of trying to cope entirely alone.

Balance is what it is all about, balancing the good things from the large families with the individual care of the smaller ones, then you'll find that living together can and does work, for all the members of the family.

LIVING ALONE

Most people, at one time or another during their lifetime, will live alone. Certainly the problems of living together with other people can be just as difficult, but they are different. Being alone all the time creates a special kind of stress, whether you are young and not yet married, middle-aged and divorced, or an older widow adjusting to life without a husband.

In general, the problems come from the fact that all the responsibility for everyday life falls only on one pair of shoulders – yours! If the plumbing breaks down, if a meal has to be prepared, if you want to see friends, go to a movie, buy a ticket, or play tennis, the effort to make these things happen must come from you, and you alone. There is no one to help you decide what to do, no one there for all the unimportant, almost silly routines which most of us take for granted.

On the positive side, though, if you can manage to cope reasonably well with the small things, then you can learn to put the larger problems in perspective, and explore some of the benefits of living alone.

Here are some of the areas which can cause a lot of stress, and a few hints on how to deal with them.

Eating alone
One of the worst culprits, and a hazard to the health of every single-person household is the problem of making sure you get enough of the right kind of food. All too often it seems easier to open a packet of starchy crackers or eat another bar of chocolate instead of preparing a good meal. It may be possible to get along quite happily like that for a while, but sooner or later your health will suffer.

You need just as much nourishment as a family member – being alone does not give you an extra quota of vitamins or minerals. So make sure you shop regularly every week, and keep the cupboard stocked with healthy, nutritious snacks. If you are going to snatch a meal on the run, at least it should be made up of good bread, cheese and salad.

Try to set aside one afternoon during the weekend to prepare a few dinners for the next week. Freeze them in one-meal quantities, and pop them in the oven as you need them. Concentrate on things you enjoy, and make sure that you treat yourself like a guest, to be tempted with new recipes and unusual dishes. Then when you do have a party you'll be able to make something different.

Try and keep to some sort of schedule so you're not tempted to skip meals too often. Watching a special television show every night can help.

Treat yourself to dinner out occasionally. If you have a good local restaurant, learn to know when it isn't too crowded, so you won't feel isolated in a sea of chatter. Waiters often take special care of people who are alone, and nowadays women as well as men can enjoy a good meal and a glass of beer or wine without feeling as if they are outcasts.

Sleeping late

A frequent problem of living alone is trying to find the right amount of sleep for yourself. It's very easy to be tempted to stay up very late watching television or reading – there's no one to remind you that the alarm clock will go off at a very early hour the next morning. The exact opposite can happen at the weekends, when you don't have to go to work, and the impulse to stay in bed can be overwhelming. Sleeping until noon may be fine for movie stars; for most of us it disrupts the whole day, as we rush around trying madly to get everything done before the shops close, still groggy and half-awake. Too much sleep is as bad as too little.

Make a schedule for yourself, based on how many hours you need to feel your best, and try to get to bed most evenings at the same time, and get up at a reasonable hour.

Exercise and sport

Exercising alone can also be a problem if you enjoy a game which needs two people all the time. Try to find a regular partner who is free when you are, and if it needs planning, like booking a tennis court, then book in advance for a number of weeks so you won't be tempted to let it go because you're too busy! You'll have to take the initiative and make more elaborate plans now and then, but that can be lots of fun. Get away for a skiing week, join a dance club or a gym with a squash court. And try to get enthusiastic about at least one sport you can practice on your own when your partner isn't able to join you – running, swimming, ballet, gymnastics – they can be very enjoyable as well as getting you out of the house regularly.

Loneliness

Everyone is lonely at one time or another, and it is always painful. People who live alone often don't have too much choice as to whether or not they have company. Sharing whatever you do every minute of the day can be unhealthy. Use your time well, read the books you've put off since your schooldays, go to concerts no one else is interested in, or just let yourself think now and then without interruption.

Remember that there is nothing lonelier than two people who can't communicate with each other, but who live in the same house; count your blessings, and learn to treasure your solitude.

A FEW SPECIAL POINTERS

- Make sure someone else has a set of keys to your home, as well as the address and phone number of your nearest relatives. Accidents do happen.

- Learn to be a little more assertive, and don't expect other people to call you all the time just because you are alone. Take the initiative, invite friends for drinks, ask them to join you for a meal or an outing, and pay your share!

- Sometimes not having to think about anyone else can lead to a selfish life; try to do something regularly about helping other people cope with *their* problems. Baby-sit for a cousin, volunteer to work at a local hospital once a month, get interested in a charity or a school. You'll find you enjoy helping other people, and you'll help yourself.

261

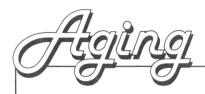

AS YEARS GO BY

Aging is universal. Sooner or later every living thing gets old. But how and when it happens is highly individual. This depends on genetic inheritance and general fitness, plus one's life-style and even how one thinks about aging. But more than anything else, it depends on use and disuse.

Until recently it was assumed that as people got older they naturally became mentally less acute, physically weaker and somewhat depressed emotionally. Studies show that these things are far from inevitable and depend mostly on whether or not, as the years go by, you have continued to make use of all your capacities, from the muscles in your limbs, to the memory-storing functions of your brain. If throughout your life you can continue to exercise mental, emotional and physical abilities, you will age more slowly, retain your clarity of mind longer, and probably remain physically and mentally fit until death ends a long and fulfilling life.

Few people realise this important truth. Most of us take a rather fatalistic view of aging, wrongly believing that there is nothing we can do about it and looking forward only to loneliness, chronic illness, senility. What really does await you in later years also depends on your expectations. If you *expect* to become senile, you probably will. Gerentologists now know that a 75 year-old can have all the symptoms of senility, although his brain cells with reveal none of the physical changes that accompany real senility. Happily, studies of old people also show that these symptoms can be eliminated by helping the patient to develop new mental and physical skills and a renewed interest in people and things outside himself.

One person's sixty is another's forty. Not chronological, but mental and biological age are what counts. And these age labels *can* be self-determined and adjusted.

On a biological level, the aging of your body is thought to be the result of loss of cells and a decline in the ability of the remaining cells to function properly. Among the things which scientists believe play an important part in the degenerative process are: radiation wastes and pollutants in the body, loss of the body's ability to differentiate between its own proteins and foreign ones that lead to deterioration of the connective tissue, and changes in the cells' genetic code which means that new cells no longer accurately resemble the earlier cells from which they were made.

There are also many theories about how from a purely physical point of view, you can slow down this degenerative process. How much one eats may also be important. Cultures such as the Vilcabamba Indians, the Abkhasians and Hunzas – known for their health and longevity – all consume a diet much lower in calories than we do in the West. They also consume less animal fat and have lower cholesterol levels. Many experts believe that air pollution also plays a large part in aging by bringing about degenerative changes in the cells, and by now everyone knows that prolonged exposure to the sun will age the skin itself far more quickly than anything else. Caffeine in coffee, drugs, alcohol and nicotine speed up aging too. But just as important as the physical 'agers' are a person's mental attitude and social relationships. Long-lived societies have a well-developed social order where as many as four generations live together, each with a sense of having something valuable to contribute to the welfare of the others. In our Western culture obsessed with youth, old people are often treated as a source of embarrassment instead of being treasured for their experience which they'd only be too happy to share with younger generations. This leads to a sense of worthlessness which is high on the list of mental attitudes that cause early aging. Human beings need to know that they can contribute something to their community and their society. Without this, the wasting process is rapid and inevitable.

In our society, we must make sure this doesn't happen to us for no-one is likely to do it for us. This means planning early for retirement, and ensuring that at each stage in your life you go on making constant use of your mind. It also means relationships with people. That includes sex, too. The human body goes on responding to affection as long as mind and body are working. For it is only through use that you can prevent deterioration. And its never too late to start. Many a flabby 60-year-old has eased himself into an exercise regime and in a few months' time emerged fitter, healthier and sexier than he's been for fifteen years.

Checklist For A Long And Happy Life

- Keep your mind active and clear by learning new things.

- Act your physio-logical age, don't launch into a strenuous exercise routine if you're flabby. Ease into it instead. On the other hand, if you are fit, don't let yourself go to pot.

- Don't look ahead to retirement as an end. Instead plan for it by developing – long beforehand – a second career or skill that you will be able to pursue. Take more education. People need to learn to retire: It is an art and when done well can be a source of great satisfaction and a time of freedom to explore new areas of life and living.

- Companionship and sex are even more important when there are fewer people to share with. If you are married do your best to make the bond deeper and stronger. Also get out and get involved in community work and organisations where you can share with others your abilities and friendship.

- Give up smoking … the life expectancy of abstainers is six years longer than that of people who smoke 20 cigarettes a day.

- Have regular check-ups and have any health problems that arise treated promptly.

- Accept yourself and learn to live with whatever disabilities you have whether mental or physical. But don't let an idea that you are incapable of doing something keep you from trying.

263

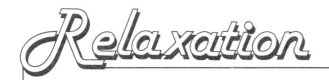

KEY TO WELL-BEING

For generations people have been saying 'Relax, it will do you good'. But only recently, thanks to in-depth research into the psychology and physiology of stress and relaxation, has anyone been able to say why. We now know prolonged excess stress – and the bodily changes it induces – can trigger many disorders, from simple insomnia to serious illness. Science also confirms that these changes are opposite in almost every way to those that occur when the body is in a state of deep relaxation. But for a long time it was assumed that, because these changes were under the control of the involuntary nervous system and therefore beyond conscious control, there was no way we could deliberately alter them.

Now we know differently. Researchers have discovered that through relaxation we can exercise a high level of control over the release of nervous tension, and that when excessive tension is in the body and is released, the physical and psychological effects of stress are significantly reduced. But the benefits of relaxation don't end there. Recent studies show that the regular periodic release of mental and physical tension also leads to improved perception; often a spontaneous decrease in dependence on alcohol, cigarettes and drugs and a generally improved mental outlook – including a greater capacity for interaction with other people and heightened creativity. One reason why so many corporations have initiated relaxation regimes for their executives.

But relaxation is rather a vague word. What does it mean? To some it means flopping in a heap on the bed. To others it brings ideas of pleasant physical activities such as golf and swimming. Of course, it is all of these things. But scientists, interested in its physical and mental benefits, take it to mean the release of unnecessary tension through the action of simply 'letting go'. To some degree we experience this when playing golf, walking in the woods, or listening to music. It results in a feeling of renewal and enjoyment, which is too often lost again soon after resuming our normal routine. But to be able to turn on such relaxation at will is an art that for most of us needs to be learnt. It is simple to do by training ourselves through specific relaxation techniques designed to release contracted muscles and overworked minds.

Once you have acquired this ability to let go you can put it to use whenever necessary. You can move at will out of the highly-active, dynamic state of action that characterizes stress, excitement and the acceptance of challenge, into the passive, receptive state of peaceful relaxation necessary for bodily regeneration, rest and creativity. You'll find that you are no longer so troubled by other people, or disturbing outside influences, and you have greater independence.

One of the funny ideas many people have about relaxation is they think it is the way we should be all the time. Another myth is that if they let themselves relax, they will lose their ambition and drive. Neither is true. Both active dynamism (stress) and creative receptivity (relaxation) are necessary in order to live fully.

Most of us 'get stuck' somewhere. Our bodies suffer, our minds become too easily clouded or confused and, in the long run, we are less than we could be. Learning to relax is an important key to getting 'unstuck'. It can also help a lot in your relationships with others. You'll find yourself getting less upset about small things, yet more able to fight for the big ones. And it will do wonders for your looks – improving posture, smoothing away lines of care and tension.

Many people who learn a technique for conscious relaxation or meditation are also amazed at how much extra energy they have. Instead of feeling worn out at the end of the day and drowning your tension and fatigue in drinks and television, try retreating alone to a room and practising your chosen technique. You'll emerge ten or twenty minutes later feeling literally a new person, able to enjoy dinner and to spend a pleasant evening with friends and family.

Relaxation is useful for slimmers too. Over-eating is often an expression of tension rather than appetite. Get rid of the tension and – coupled with a good diet it will go a long way towards getting rid of excess pounds.

Conscious relaxation, once you've mastered it, becomes easier and easier until it is almost automatic. Practised regularly, one or two exercises for relaxation will soon become personal tools you can call on every day when there is a small lull in your routine or when you need them most.

1. Relax your body to overcome fatigue and quickly refresh yourself.

2. Relax your mind and body when you feel anger, frustration, disappointment.

3. Relax to reduce your blood pressure if you suffer from hypertension.

4. Relax to increase bodily circulation sending nutrients to the body's cells and carrying away wastes, when you feel the first signs of a cold or flu. (In some cases deep relaxation used like this can actually ward off the trouble before it begins.)

5. Relax your body and mind before beginning any project that demands clarity of thought.

6. Relax to decrease muscle tension and help eliminate the aches and pains that crop up particularly in the shoulders and back or to get rid of a headache without having to take aspirin.

7. Relax when you are late for an appointment, caught in traffic or having to wait somewhere … in short whenever you are in irritating circumstances which you cannot control. It can actually turn a nightmare of tension and frustration into a pleasant time for contemplation.

8. Relax regularly to decrease your dependence on cigarettes, alcohol, or too much food.

9. Relax to give you quick and lasting energy. To make you feel stronger, more confident and to improve your all-round fitness.

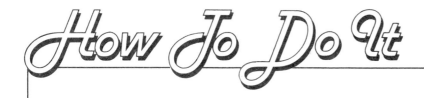

THREE RELAXATION TECHNIQUES

There are many different techniques you can use to relax. Experiment with a few until you find the ones that suit you best. Remember that one may work best for you when you are lying in bed, while another is better when you are sitting in a bus, or a train.

Muscle Awareness Technique is particularly good for making you understand how to control the tension in your muscles deliberately, so you learn to recognize the signs before you become too tense to relax at all.

The Relaxation Response quietens the mind while it helps to relieve the stresses of a long day. Self-directed Total Body Relaxation is the perfect tool for all-over tiredness, when you need to get up refreshed and revitalized within a few minutes.

Try them all, and see what each can do for you.

MUSCLE AWARENESS TECHNIQUE

Often used as part of the training of women for natural childbirth, this tool is ideal for getting rid of all the aches and pains which are the result of unconscious tension in muscles. To eliminate tension you must first become aware of it and of the difference in feeling between relaxed muscles and tensed ones.

Scientific research confirms that when there is no excess muscle tension, the mind becomes calm as well, so this exercise is also a useful way of calming anxiety, and relieving depression. It takes about ten minutes to do and it's best to practise it a couple of times a day, perhaps on waking, while you're still in bed, and again just before dinner to make you fresh for the evening. It can be done either sitting comfortably in a chair or lying on a firm bed or the floor. (A soft bed is not good as it makes it easy to hang on to tension without realising it).

1. Make yourself comfortable either lying flat with a cushion under your knees with or without a pillow under your head, or sitting in an easy chair with your back well supported and your feet on the floor. Make sure you are warm enough. (When the body relaxes, the temperature drops slightly). If you are not covered with a blanket or shawl, you'll get cold.

Close your eyes. Take two or three deep breaths.

2. Tense your whole body, tightening every muscle of every part as much as possible. Now slowly relax, focusing your attention on

each part of your body in turn as you relax it, beginning with your feet and working all the way up to your head. Pay particular attention to your abdomen, chest, shoulders, jaw and neck.

3. Do the same again, but this time tense up your body only half as much as you did before. Then slowly, consciously, let go of each part in turn from toe to head.

4. Repeat the exercise, but this time tense your body only just enough to give a *slight* feeling of tension, no more. Now release each part until there is a sensation of relaxation all over, passing your attention over each part of the body in turn.

5. Now focus on your arms only, bending your elbow, making a fist and bringing it up to your chest so both arms are hard with muscle tension. As you do this, check to see that all the rest of your body remains relaxed. The tension should only be in your arms and hands, nowhere else. Let go. Breathe deeply.

6. Now tighten up both legs at the same time, making every muscle hard. Check to see that the rest of your body remains relaxed. Now let go with everything.

7. Practise the same thing with each arm and leg in turn, tightening the muscles then letting go, all the while checking that the rest of you remains relaxed. Try tensing opposite arms and legs together. Then release, until you are able to isolate tension in the part of your body you choose, and then let it go at will. After several practice sessions you will immediately sense when part of your body is tense during the day. Then all you need do to relax it is exaggerate the tension as much as

possible, checking that the rest of you remains relaxed, and give the mental order to let go.

8. Finish off each practice session with a dozen gentle deep breaths. Open your eyes, giving yourself a moment to 'come back' before you get up.

RELAXATION RESPONSE

Developed by Harvard cardiologist Herbert Benson MD, this technique is simple, and once you have the hang of it you can do it practically anywhere … a park bench, an office (provided you take the telephone off the hook) or even a commuter train. All you need to begin with is a quiet environment, a chair to sit on and regular practice.

Here's how:

1. *Choose a quiet place.* Your office will be fine if you can be sure you won't be interrupted for about 20 minutes, or a quiet room at home.

2. *Find yourself a comfortable position.* Sit in a comfortable chair, preferably one with a straight back, so the base of your spine is well supported and you can breathe fully and freely. (Lying down is not a good idea because we tend to associate this position with sleep, rather than alertness that comes with conscious relaxation of this kind). When you're in position, gently sway back and forth a couple of times to 'settle in'. Then quietly take a few deep breaths.

3. *Pick yourself a mental tool.* It can be a sound that you like or a word like 'one' or 'peace', an image that pleases you such as a flower or a place, or simply thinking of a person that makes you happy. Then close your eyes and visualise in the 'mind's eye' your object or place, or repeat the sound or word to yourself.

4. *Cultivate a passive turning away from everyday thoughts.* Whenever an ordinary thought intrudes, gently turn your mind back to your image or sound. Don't worry about it, this kind of distraction is normal and won't interfere with the effectiveness of the technique. Gradually, with practice, the whole process will become easier and easier. (It is something that is done without effort anyway).

5. *Practise regularly.* Go through this routine for twenty minutes twice a day.

SELF-DIRECTED TOTAL BODY RELAXATION

This is an excellent exercise for becoming aware of the amazing powers of self-suggestion because the technique is accomplished completely through directions given by your mind. It requires no physical effort. The whole process takes about ten minutes and should be practised twice a day.

Sit comfortably in a chair with your lower back supported and feet on the floor, or lie flat on a firm surface with a pillow under your head and another just under the knees so that they are slightly bent and your thighs fall outwards a little. Arms are at your sides or lightly resting on your lap. Close your eyes. Slowly take five deep breaths, letting the air out completely each time. Then breathe normally.

First think about your feet. Forget everything else. Now mentally tell your feet to relax. Say to yourself, 'my feet are relaxing, getting heavy and loose'. Now move on to your ankles, 'my ankles are getting loose and floppy, I let them go completely'. Now go on to your calves, 'my calves are getting loose and heavy. I relax them completely'. Now give the same directions to your thighs, your hips, making yourself aware of that part of your body only, forgetting the rest with each suggestion. Now go on to your back, your abdomen, your shoulders, your arms, hands and fingers. Finally move your awareness to your head and face. 'I relax my head, it sinks peacefully and pleasantly into the pillow. Every muscle of my face is going soft and relaxed. My jaw is relaxed, my eyes are relaxed, my tongue, my lips, my forehead, my whole head is completely relaxed.' Now finish off the whole body with, 'my whole body is completely still, warm, relaxed and at peace. I can feel it in my mind'.

Now count backwards from ten, relaxing the whole more and more with each number. 'Ten, I am warm and peaceful, so calm and relaxed. Nine, I let go more … more … more; eight, more … more … more … and so on down to one. By this time you will be deeply relaxed and feel healthy and calm. Now be still for a couple of minutes, breathing deeply and savouring the pleasant sensation of peace and calm all through you. When you want to finish, say to yourself. 'Now I am going to open my eyes and get up feeling pleasantly fresh and well'. Open your eyes and slowly get up.

The secret of success with this exercise is perseverance. At first it might be difficult. You may find it hard to be aware of the sensations of relaxation. But you should remember that your feet, legs, hips and whole body *are* relaxing. After practising several times you will begin to feel the sensations of relaxation as warmth, tingling, pulsing in different areas of your body. Remember the whole routine needs no physical effort, the relaxation comes through your body as a result of the mental suggestion you are giving it. Try not to *do* anything. Just let it happen.

OTHER METHODS OF LETTING GO

Here are some useful relaxing and energising tricks (some *both* at the same time) drawn from traditional yoga techniques. They can be done quickly and take effect in a few moments.

1 *Energy breath*
   Great for when you are feeling drowsy from inactivity or over-tired. Exhale as deeply and fully as you can, then take a deep breath from the abdomen. Exhale again immediately through the nose, jerking in your abdomen quickly so it pushes the air out forcefully. Relax the abdomen and then jerk in again, expelling more air. Repeat this five times until the lungs are completely empty. Now take in a long slow breath, retain it for a count of five and slowly let it all out. Repeat the whole exercise five times. (If you feel giddy, stop. Never overstrain).

2 *The decanter*
   To still an over-active mind.
   Sit comfortably. Imagine your body as a decanter with the bottom of the decanter being your hips and abdomen, and that you are going to fill the decanter with energy. Now breathe in slowly, imagining that it is becoming full. When you've taken in as much air as you can and you are 'getting to the top', hold your breath long enough to become aware of your own fullness. Now exhale slowly and imagine that the bottle is emptying. Repeat five to ten times. If you find you become a little light-headed, don't worry, it is normal.

3 *Prana power*
   This is a way of using air to help get rid of minor aches and pains caused by tension, a simple yogic technique for directing air energy or 'prana' to different parts of the body where it is needed. It takes only a few minutes to do. Sitting in a relaxed and comfortable position, breathe in slowly and deeply, visualising the life energy you are taking in. Hold your breath for a few seconds, then as you breathe out visualise sending the energy from the air you've breathed in into the particular party of the body you want to affect, imagining it as you *want* it to be, (ie. soft, tension-free muscles in the shoulders, a smooth cool forehead, etc.). Repeat for from three to five minutes at a time.

DE-TENSERS

Muscle tension is often the major cause of excess fatigue and aches and pains for office workers. Here are a few easy-to-do relaxation techniques for immediate results. These De-tensers can take only five minutes and can be done at a desk or standing in an office. They need no huffing and puffing. But there's a bonus to them too ... while they are making you unwind they'll also help tone you up and slim you down.

1 *For neck and face muscles:*
   Sitting up in a straight-backed chair, drop your head backwards, letting your jaw fall open. Now bite down on an imaginary apple five times, feeling the stretch in your neck and face muscles. Now, head still back, close your mouth, puff out your cheeks and draw them in again, tightly five times.

2 *For aching, tense shoulders and neck:*
   Do exaggerated shoulder shrugs ... raising them as high as possible then lowering them as far as they'll go five times. Rotate one shoulder at a time in a circle, first forward and then back, three times each. Now do the other shoulder. Next let the head fall forward rotating it to the side, back, and the other side, letting the weight of your head move itself. Make three circles one way, then three the other, keeping your eyes closed.

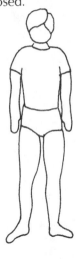

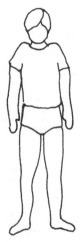

3 *All-over Energizer:*
   Sitting straight, feet on floor, hands on
   knees, arch your back, letting the head fall
   backwards. Now contract in your middle,
   tightening tummy muscles, dropping the
   head forwards, bending elbows and
   curving torso over. Finally uncurl very
   slowly bringing your head up last, with
   shoulders loose and tummy muscles held
   in. Repeat slowly five times.

4 *For legs and feet;*
   Sitting with arms parallel reaching forward
   at shoulder level, kick one leg straight out
   in front of you and flex the foot backwards
   and forwards ten times. Now repeat with
   the other foot.

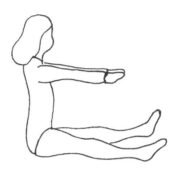

5 *The great loosener*
   Standing, feet 18 inches apart and parallel,
   with back straight, bend at the hips, letting
   head, shoulders and arms fall forward.
   Stay there for 30 seconds to one minute,
   then slowly uncurl. Repeat twice.

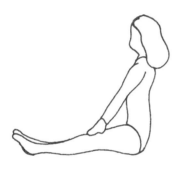

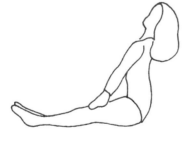

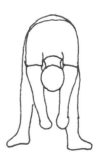

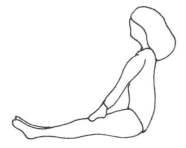

6 Thigh stretch

Start with your feet in a "V". Then go up on your toes and bend the knees very slowly till you you reach the final position above. This is an especially difficult exercise and you shouldn't tackle it till you've been practising a while. Good for ankles.

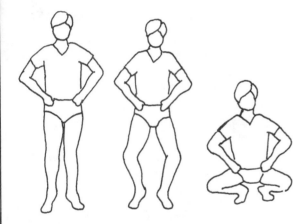

7 The swan posture

A wonderful way to relax and at the same time it's good for your back and straightening your spine. Simply lie down with your arms over ... just like a swan in fact.

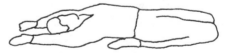

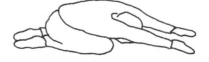

Meditation

MEDITATION AND AWARENESS

At its simplest level, meditation is a very special method of relaxation, teaching you to let go, and allowing your mind to become completely still, serene and receptive.

Its benefits include the power to combat stress and tiredness, it increases your physical and mental energy, and it can even treat medical conditions such as raised blood pressure, migraine, and tension headaches. Meditation can also increase a feeling of stability and serenity, especially important in our complex world where so many of us live with a feeling of nervousness and tension so much of the day.

The teachers of meditation say that such a state of mind also makes it possible to understand the true nature of consciousness and reality, although even the desire to reach that state must be given up before it can happen. This is meditation at its most profound level, practised for itself without expectations of any kind, entirely for its own sake.

There are many different schools of meditation, and they have different techniques and ways of achieving the same result. You can begin with "mindfulness of breathing" which you learn by counting your breath, and becoming aware of the air coming in and going out of your body.

TRANSCENDENTAL MEDITATION

The mantra meditation (Transcendental Meditation or TM is the best known) uses a word or a syllable repeated continuously. You can be alone or in a group, speak silently or in your mind, the intention is to clear the surface of the mind of all mental activity.

You may choose to meditate on a particular subject such as compassion or death, or on an object – a flower, a candle, or an image held in your own mind, or on a particular part of the body such as the tip of your nose or the traditional choice, the navel.

There is also the simple observation of standing back and observing your thoughts as they come and go, or thinking about a visual pattern which moves and changes – a rose opening, a butterfly in flight. There are some forms of Yoga, and the formless meditation of Zen. These are only a few of the many methods which can expand your conscious awareness and clear your mind of unimportant trivia.

In many ways, elementary meditation closely resembles deep relaxation – the techniques bring about the same changes in brain wave patterns, a marked decrease in the rate of breathing and the consumption of oxygen, an improved memory and better concentration.

If you are basically interested in learning to cope with conflicts and stresses in your life so that you can be healthier and fitter, then one of the relaxation exercises or any one of the meditation methods would probably work.

If you want to explore the philosophy behind each system, then read about each method and judge for yourself if it seems to offer you an expanding world within yourself. Whatever you choose, remember that the great teachers of meditation and religion have said that all roads lead sooner or later to the same place.

DO-IT-YOURSELF ZAZEN

If you would like to try a meditational technique on your own, here is a well-tried and proven one (several thousands of years old) without philosophical or religious overtones. Although it involves breathing, it is not a breathing exercise. It is an exercise in awareness. You are merely using the breath as it enters and leaves the body as a focus for your attention. This after a little practice has the effect of releasing the mind and relaxing the body.

Here's how:

Find a quiet place and seat yourself comfortably in a chair with your spine supported well, or cross-legged on the floor. Close your eyes. Take two or three breaths, letting out your air completely each time to relax. Now you are ready to begin! As you breathe in and out, count after each breath silently to yourself until you reach the tenth breath, and then go back and start again. So it goes like this: in-breath … out-breath … one … in-breath … out-breath … two … in-breath … out-breath … three … and so on. If you lose track of the count don't worry, just go back to one and begin again, breathing naturally all the while. The object of the meditation is neither to get to ten nor to control or change your breathing in any way. Just be aware of it as it comes in through your nose and then goes out again. That's all. Continue for fifteen minutes. Practise the technique twice a day for a couple of weeks and you should be pleasantly surprised at the results.

What to do about distractions (such as remembering the appointment you have tomorrow or thoughts like 'this is silly'): Nothing. They are normal and don't interfere with the effectiveness of the meditation at all. Simply bring your attention *gently* (the gently is important as the mind can never be forced) back to your breath and the counting.

Getting the most from all kinds of leisure depends on good planning, a strong dose of good sense and good humour. Vacations should provide a complete change of pace that breaks all the usual habits of your ordinary life and lifts you out of the rut. So if you have to drive all day in your job, choose the sort of holiday where there isn't too much driving involved. If you have to cook every day for the family, you might convince everyone to stay at a guest house or a hotel where the cooking and cleaning are done for you. Mothers in particular often get forgotten. If you're still going to do housework, even in a foreign city, make out some kind of rota so the work will be shared.

Of course, the ideal holiday is not always possible, either because of finances, or because your own idea of a perfect two weeks away might be very different from the rest of the family. But there are so many choices today – don't just give up – packages for sightseeing as well as resident courses for all kinds of special interests from archaeology to zither-playing! This is a time for compromise. If one year you agree to someone else's dream of camping beside a mountain stream, then decide together as a family that the next year you will all do something *you* would enjoy.

It makes sense to choose a less expensive trip and have enough money left to spend just for fun than be right up to your financial limits and have to worry about it all the time. Plan the travel carefully too. If you drive, leave enough time and don't plan to go too far each day, otherwise you will end up more exhausted on your return than before you left.

Once you get there, remember that change of any kind may upset people physically, especially children – different food, water, surroundings, routines and noises. It takes a few days to settle in. Give yourself time and don't make the mistake of eating and drinking far too much.

Hobbies and sports need the same careful planning. The first and most vital question to ask yourself is simple: do I really enjoy it or has it become a habit? Do I really love knitting argyle socks or would it be more fun to build furniture? Or take photographs? Leisure time should bring you all the valuable rest and relaxation you need, away from responsibilities of day-to-day problems. And enjoyment is important for its own sake, not just a kind of self-indulgence. It's an essential part of staying fit and healthy. Pleasure calms the mind and the nervous system, eliminates feelings of strain, and helps relax those chronically tense muscles. Even grown-ups need playtime – to explore the most rewarding and creative ideas, and simply to have fun.

CHOOSING THE RIGHT HOBBY FOR YOU

Here are a few questions to ask yourself about hobbies and leisure activities. If most of your answers are 'yes', you're well matched and probably getting as much relaxation and mental stimulation as you need. If most of your answers are 'no', why not look around at some new possibilities? Join a class, read a book, open your eyes to what is around you.

1. Do the activities you like best provide:
   (a) As complete a physical change from work as possible? So if your job is sedentary, your leisure activities are physically demanding?
   (b) As complete a change of environment as possible so you are in a different place, dressed differently and preferably with different people too?
   (c) Do you enjoy your hobby because it's fun, no matter how badly you do it, or do you think it's only worth while if you do it extremely well and win, too? This is a very important point – the ambitious person with drive and a strong competitive spirit should try to relax with a non-competitive hobby – you can become just as strained and anxious about a golf club championship as you are about getting that new account at the office. Variety is the spice of life.
2. Did you discover some of your leisure activities by yourself, or were you persuaded by your doctor or a member of your family that you ought to enjoy them?
3. Do you feel happier and more relaxed from day to day after a few leisure hours or do you carry your anxieties with you?
4. Do you set aside enough time for yourself, and what you enjoy doing, knowing that leisure is a valuable and important part of good health, or do you let yourself get sidetracked by problems and unnecessary work?
5. Do you get at least an hour or two a week of strenuous exercise (running, swimming, tennis, squash, football etc.)? Or if your job involves a great deal of hard physical work, do you get a few hours of restful leisure a week – that keeps your mind active instead of your body?
6. Can you make yourself do something interesting now and then instead of watching television all the time?
7. Do you realize that the rest of the family needs to explore their own interests quite apart from you? This goes for children as well as adults.
8. Do you ever really let yourself have fun? Do something that's a bit crazy, just to break the routine? Let yourself get away long enough to just be like a child for a while ... free, and maybe even a bit foolish?

A FEW SUGGESTIONS

If you are	Why not try this?
Non-domestic, highly competitive, mentally active and strung up all day ...	Unusual kinds of cooking, embroidery, fine cabinet making, listening to new music, painting.
housebound, physically tired out but mentally dulled by routine or young children ...	Go to yoga class, plan and build a new garden, join a dramatic club, a dancing class, take up rock collecting, writing and poetry, making pottery.

Stress in Your Life

THE PROBLEMS OF EVERY DAY LIFE

Stress is a fact of life, neither good nor bad. If you learn to make use of it, it will help you feel and think clearly, and fill you with one exciting challenge after another day by day. If you let it make use of you, you will be exhausted, unable to think and act decisively, or even seriously ill.

You can put stress on your body through the physical demands you make on yourself. Mental stress comes from drastic or prolonged shifts of emotion either from negative feelings such as worry, frustration or unhappiness, or from positive feelings such as profound joy, excitement or love. The senses of our minds and bodies can never be really separated; they always occur together.

The body reacts to all stress in exactly the same way, equiping us to deal with the extra demands. When faced with an emergency situation such as the threat of being fired, the joy of reunion or simply loud and prolonged noise, adrenal secretions flash into the blood, bringing strength in the form of fat and sugar energy to the brain and muscles. The pulse races, blood pressure and cholesterol levels rise and breathing becomes faster. Much of the blood supply to the internal organs is immediately redirected into the muscles which become ready for physical action so the body can mobilize all its energies to fight or to run away – the 'red alert' state.

Within a few minutes, the body's full energy potential has been realized. We take some sort of action, and then the secretions stop. The adrenalin is burnt off, the sugar and fat are used up, the blood flow returns to its general duties of supplying all the internal organs and systems that keep the body in healthy running order.

At least, that's how it *should* work. The trouble is that modern high-pressured life surrounds us with almost constant threats that unconsciously trigger off our 'red alert' response.

Thousands of years ago, quick and decisive action would solve the problems of wild animals or physical danger, and at the same time it burnt off all the extra chemicals our bodies produced. Today, we rarely have any physical outlet, we swallow our frustration, apparently remain calm and undisturbed, and these substances accumulate in the body along with the physical and emotional tension that accompanies them. It builds and builds until many of us live in a permanently stressed state, unable to come down again to peace and relaxation.

This is where stress becomes dangerous. Unusual amounts of adrenalin can be stored in the heart where it affects its functioning, increasing the heartbeat rate even when the body is at rest, decreasing its ability to use oxygen and causing irregularities. Excess stress contributes to feelings of fatigue and depression. In prolonged stress, there is also an unconscious tensing of muscles.

Stress is now linked with heart disease, arthritis, ulcers, high-blood pressure, constricted blood vessels, and mental disorders. These are the negative aspects of excess stress.

278

But there are important positive aspects too. An occasional shot of adrenalin is a great cure for boredom and indifference. We often do our best when we are under some stress. But beyond a certain level, which is different for each individual, stress becomes destructive. Get to know how much stress you need to make you perform just that little bit better, but before it becomes damaging and unhealthy.

MAKING IT WORK FOR YOU

Everyone reacts differently to that 'red alert'; stress. Some find great stress and even danger a great pleasure, for others it's simply too much to cope with. A few even become addicted to stress dependent upon high levels of stress hormones such as adrenaline and noradrenalin in the system instead of to nicotine or alcohol. They live with prolonged high levels of stress for so long, it seems normal. This can be serious. For example business tycoons and pop stars can suffer from being stress-aholics, and it's very hard to go back to normal everyday life.

Cigarettes and alcohol are not the answer either. Both bring about many of the same physiological changes in the body as stress itself. Nicotine, for instance, raises blood pressure, the heart beat rate and levels of stress hormones and cholesterol. While smoking and drinking may seem to help for the time being, they are actually contributing to the stress overload problem in the long run.

But when stress is handled well, it gives us added motivation to overcome obstacles, and an ideal warning system that brings awareness and strength to handle threatening situations that might damage or destroy our happiness, safety and self-esteem. The ability to work under pressure is an important asset.

Don't try to avoid stress altogether – use it instead. Every crisis offers an opportunity to let the adrenalin work. Take some kind of action to burn up that extra stress-energy – make a decision, hit the ball hard, scrub a floor very hard, run around the garden fast, and when the crisis is over, learn to forget it and relax.

Excess tension can be eliminated with amazing ease, once you develop a tool for conscious relaxation and use it regularly. Deep relaxation and stress are like two sides of a coin; each is the exact opposite of the other in the physiological and mental changes it brings about. They complement each other like light and dark, summer and winter. Learn to move from one to the other and you have a key to success in almost everything you try. Sounds simple? It is.

Tranquillizers are not the best solution to continual stress; the longer you take them the less effective they become. There are serious side effects, too, so try not to rely on pills too much.

HOW STRESSED ARE YOU?

Here is a questionnaire to help you assess your own level of general stress and become aware of any 'problem' areas you may have. It is simple to do. Pick out the statement in each category which best describes you in the particular situation. In some cases you may find that two statements describe you, but pick the one that comes closest to how you usually react or causes you the most difficulty.

1. When playing a competitive sport do you:
   - ☐ (a) find yourself wasting energy through tension and anxiety?
   - ☐ (b) assume you will do well and throw yourself into the game without much worry about whether you win or lose?
   - ☐ (c) worry about how your performance may be viewed by others?
   - ☐ (d) need to win at all costs and suffer profound disappointment if you don't?

2. When driving in heavy traffic do you:
   - ☐ (a) remain calm, alert and relaxed and take delays as a matter of course?
   - ☐ (b) find your heart beating faster and feel irritated about the delay?
   - ☐ (c) find yourself getting actively angry with other motorists and want them to get out of your way even if it means driving too fast or carelessly.
   - ☐ (d) become tired and worried about the time being wasted?

3. When meeting new people at work or a social event, do you:
   - ☐ (a) feel relaxed and face the meeting with a sense of excitement because there might be something new and wonderful about them?
   - ☐ (b) become tense, find your heart pounding and hands becoming sweaty?
   - ☐ (c) worry about how they will think about you and fear that you may say something awkward or foolish?
   - ☐ (d) find yourself becoming bored and listless?

4. When you wake up in the morning, how do you feel:
   - ☐ (a) alert and happy, looking forward to the day ahead?
   - ☐ (b) anxious, with lots of different thoughts about what you have to do rushing through your head?

(c) hoping desperately that the day ahead will hold something of interest to you?

(d) not too bad, but resigned to the fact that each day is much like any other … nothing wonderful is going to happen?

5. When demanding what you want from a business colleague, friend or marriage partner, do you:

(a) feel it is too much of an effort to pursue your demands when you meet the first signs of opposition?

(b) try to convince yourself you shouldn't feel too strongly about anything.

(c) forcefully insist that this is what you are going to have or do without regard for their objections or ideas?

(d) enter into the confrontation eager to state your side of things, listen to theirs and relatively confident the two of you can come to a mutual agreement with a little give and take?

6. When planning a piece of work, or organizing a fairly complex event at work or home, do you usually:

(a) easily and quietly gather together all the necessary materials and facts and proceed to sort them out?

(b) find it difficult to get started because it all seems too much of an effort?

(c) become tense and uncomfortable, unsure that you will be able to handle it all?

(d) treat it all as a matter of course, preparing yourself well and then carrying out the task easily and effectively?

7. When having to deal with children's questions and difficulties, do you:

(a) become quickly irritable?

(b) find yourself bored and uninterested?

(c) dismiss them as fast and curtly as possible?

(d) listen wholeheartedly and then do everything possible to help them handle the problem effectively?

8. When a child does something you don't like, how do you react?

(a) calmly tell him you prefer him to behave differently?

(b) find it hard to summon up the energy to do anything about it?

☐ (c) feel confused and at a loss about what you should do?

☐ (d) find your temper rising and fly off the handle easily?

9. When after a long day you get in bed ready to go to sleep, do you find:

☐ (a) thoughts keep racing through your head and you become more wide awake as the minutes pass?

☐ (b) you can relax and drift off easily?

☐ (c) you toss and turn and have trouble relaxing your muscles?

☐ (d) you don't feel tired.

10. Do you feel you respond effectively to the challenges life presents you?

☐ (a) almost always.
☐ (b) rarely.
☐ (c) usually
☐ (d) almost never.

11. Do you smoke:

☐ (a) not ever.
☐ (b) less than 10 cigarettes a day.
☐ (c) less than 20 cigarettes a day.
☐ (d) more than 20 cigarettes a day.

12. What is your alcohol intake:

☐ (a) Frequent (every day) and heavy (more than four glasses of wine or three mixed drinks).

☐ (b) frequent but not heavy.

☐ (c) occasional, you drink a little, not more than three days a week.

☐ (d) light, only the rarest glass of something or nothing at all.

NOTE: SEE BOTTOM OF NEXT PAGE FOR SCORING

STRESS CHECK SCORING:

Question 1	(a)	− 2	Question 7	(a)	− 4
	(b)	+ 5		(b)	− 2
	(c)	− 1		(c)	− 3
	(d)	− 4		(d)	+ 5
Question 2	(a)	+ 5	Question 8	(a)	+ 5
	(b)	− 1		(b)	− 1
	(c)	− 4		(c)	− 2
	(d)	− 3		(d)	− 4
Question 3	(a)	+ 5	Question 9	(a)	− 4
	(b)	− 4		(b)	+ 5
	(c)	− 2		(c)	− 2
	(d)	− 1		(d)	− 1
Question 4	(a)	+ 5	Question 10	(a)	+ 5
	(b)	− 3		(b)	− 2
	(c)	− 2		(c)	+ 3
	(d)	− 1		(d)	− 4
Question 5	(a)	− 2	Question 11	(a)	+ 5
	(b)	− 1		(b)	+ 2
	(c)	− 4		(c)	+ 1
	(d)	+ 5		(d)	− 4
Question 6	(a)	+ 4	Question 12	(a)	− 4
	(b)	− 1		(b)	− 2
	(c).	− 3		(c)	+ 1
	(d)	+ 5		(d)	+ 5

HOW DID YOU SCORE?

If you scored more than + 58, you are wonderfully free of excess stress and cope very well with day to day challenges. Congratulations.

If you scored between + 26–57, you are above average in being free of excessive stress.

If you scored between − 7 to + 25, your stress load is too much although you are still within the 'safe' zone, provided you don't have to face too many serious changes in your life all at once.

If you scored below − 8, you are definitely overstressed. Try making use of all the exercise techniques and relaxation tools in this book to improve your resistance to what could become damaging prolonged strain.

STRESS, PERSONALITY AND HEART DISEASE

Two American experts on heart disease, Dr. Meyer Friedman and Dr. Ray Rosenman, have correlated personality type with the incidence of heart disease and one's ability to cope with stress. Answer the questions below, rating yourself on a scale of 0 to 10 (5 is considered average) to find out about yourself.

1. Are you eager to compete?
2. Would you say you have a driving forceful personality?
3. Do you strive for advancement in work or to win in sports?
4. Are you always trying to get things done quickly?
5. Do you want public recognition?
6. Do things and people easily make you angry?
7. Are you conscious of time and deadlines?
8. Are you eager for social advancement?
9. Do you accomplish many different activities?
10. Are you impatient when you get delayed or thwarted in your efforts?

If you score more than 85 on the scale, you are considered a Type A personality ... more than three times more likely to suffer a heart attack than the cooler, calmer, less competitive Type B personaltiy, which you are if you scored less than 5. Type B's also live with stress better without letting it get the best of them.

HOW WELL CAN YOU COPE WITH STRESS?

The higher you score on the following quiz, the more likely you will be able to cope with stress when it comes without letting it get the better of you.

1. Do you get at least an hour a week of strenuous exercise?
   If yes, score 4.
   If you get more than three hours a week, score another 2.
   If only half an hour, score 1.
   If you are fairly active in your work (i.e. not desk bound), score another 1.

2. How is your weight?

If you are less than ten pounds overweight, score 2.

If you are less than twenty-five pounds overweight, score 1.

If you rarely eat sugar or anything that contains it, score 3.

If you rarely eat oily or fatty foods, score 2.

If you average less alcohol than six glasses or two bottles of wine or twelve beers a week, score 1.

3. How is your ability to relax?

If you regularly practise a deep relaxation or meditation technique (see page 000) daily, score 5.

If you practice one at least three times a week, score 3.

If you lie down in the middle of the day for ten minutes or so, score another 2.

4. Do you smoke?

If you smoke less than ten cigarettes a day, score 2.

If you have not smoked at all for five years, score 1.

If you smoke pipes or cigars, score 1.

If you have never smoked, score 4.

5. How is your general health?

If you have had no illnesses in the past six months, score 1.

If you have suffered no accidents (cuts, bruises, falls etc.) in the past month, score 1.

If you feel very well in general, score 3; not good – not bad, score 1.

If you have taken no medication in the past three days (including aspirin, tranquillizers, cold remedies etc.), score 2.

6. How is your sleep and how do you feel when you get up in the morning? If in the last week you have usually slept:

Well, score 2.

Very tired, score 0.

A little groggy, score 1.

Very refreshed, score 3.

SCORING

To find out how healthy your day to day lifestyle is in terms of coping with stress, add up your score. Here is the key:

ABOVE 28 Bravo. You can feel reasonably secure provided you aren't faced with any great crises like the death of a relative or the loss of a job.

20–28 Not bad at all. You should do all right, but might consider more exercise or learning to relax daily.

9–19 You could do better, and should. Find out where your weak points lie and see what you can do to strengthen them.

0–8 Your life style is in urgent need of revising.

If your scores from all the quizzes indicate a high level of stress but a low ability to cope with it, it is a good idea to see what you can do to change your day to day living habits in order to strengthen your resistance. You may not be able to avoid the stress-producing events and circumstances, but you can do a lot to see they don't take their toll in ill-health. Try learning a deep relaxation technique and practising it daily, make sure your eating habits are good, cut down on alcohol or cigarettes.

THE TROUBLE IS ...

Doctors, religious leaders, novelists, playwrights, film-makers, poets and psychologists are all concerned with the quality of human life, and how we express ourselves and communicate with each other. Most of them would probably agree that there are three main subjects which cause more problems than anything else – money, work, and sex.

These all come up over and over again, in conversation, in books, in plays and television series, a good indication of how important they are to almost all of us.

It's not really surprising, of course – we spend a third of our lives working in order to earn money to live, and of all the human relationships, sex is possibly the most powerful and certainly the most complicated, since sexual feelings and responses are with us in some way from the time we are born to the end of our lives.

They are also mixed up together in all sorts of weird and wonderful combinations – sometimes not so wonderful, either. And when they cause problems, it is not always easy to sort out first which is the basic reason, and then what can be done to make things work a little better.

But to begin with it is important to try to untangle the knots and see the problems a little more clearly. Recognizing that there is a problem at all is the first step – too many of us go through life accepting unnecessary worries and painful situations because we feel there isn't any alternative.

Sometimes, of course, that is true. A job causes us physical or mental distress, but for a variety of reasons there is just no other work available. Or an unhappy marriage creates continual hostility – shouting at each other all the time, or sometimes even worse, bottling it all up 'for the children's sake' or because we are ashamed of admitting we made a mistake, and the thought of coping with the financial and social liabilities of living alone is more terrifying than the rows and the angry scenes. A parent or child is fatally ill; we know, they may not. Living every day with that kind of knowledge is a terrible strain, harder to bear because it cannot be shared.

Yet, there are always practical ways of making the strain easier, and other positive ideas which may not be the easy, cure-all solution we would like, but nonetheless can help us to cope just that little bit better, and live just that little bit more contentedly.

Of course there could be whole encyclopedias on each kind of problem – we all *vary* so much, and every one of us has a slightly different picture of what we need to be happy. Here we can only pinpoint some of the largest and darkest problems, those that crop up in almost everybody's life at one time or another. We hope that they will help you to see that you are not alone and that more than anything, you *can* do something to help yourself.

WORK AND YOUR JOB

We've said that a third of your life is spent working, but it's even more important than that – another few hours are probably spent wasted getting to your job and back, most of us tend to think about our jobs or the people we meet even when we are supposed to be relaxing or doing something else, and of course, if you add it all up, you probably spend your most productive years working every day, five days a week.

So there's plenty of time for conflicts and problems to arise. And they can come at any period, and at any age; the youngster who cannot get his first job because he has no experience, and can't get experience because he has never had a job, the middle-aged man who desperately wants to change his career but is afraid of the effect it will have on his wife and family, the older person who is dangerously near official retiring time, but who isn't ready mentally or financially to give up work altogether. Even if everything seems right, you're doing a job you basically enjoy and you have a fair amount of security, there are daily irritations and bottlenecks at work which can make you tense, irritable, and eventually affect the quality of your work and even the rest of your life.

To begin with, try to sit down and take a good look at yourself and your work. Usually even before we are willing to admit it, our minds are worrying away at the problems trying to find a solution before it's too late. So bring it out in the open; you really hate the factory floor, or the 9-to-5 routine in the office, or you think your boss is going to make trouble for you no matter what you do, or how well you do your job. The new management is going to cut down on staff, you can't see any way of getting ahead or out of the typing pool, or you simply don't trust your partner.

Whatever it is, face up to the fact that you *are* worried, and why. Otherwise it will gnaw away at your peace of mind, and eventually it will affect the rest of your life, too. Repressing real problems only leads more often than not to depression, and the longer you let it go buried inside you, the harder it is to realize what is causing your unhappiness, and the more difficult it becomes to do anything about it.

So now you have at least begun to think more clearly. Let's take some of the most common stresses:

You don't enjoy your work at all
It really is important to your whole attitude and even to your health. Many people are caught in jobs they don't like, although it may take years before they realize what they want to do. If fundamentally this is your problem, then don't just shrug your shoulders and give up. Do try and work out what upsets you most, and what you would prefer to do. There is no point in going from an insurance company to a publishing house if it turns out to be paper work that you hate; you'd be better off looking for a job in horticulture or as a door to door salesman. Or turning from teaching school to writing children's books if you don't like children! Many of us enjoy one kind of work when we begin adult life, but want to make a complete change when we reach middle age. Remember that with few exceptions, it is never impossible, and the sooner you start the more chance you will have to make a success of it.

Talk it over with your family if you can – wives and husbands are usually interested only in your welfare, and they should be able to give you support and encouragement. If the change is also going to mean less money and possibly less security, well, they should be part of the decision as well. If you do end up feeling that practical considerations mean you stay where you are, try setting a goal for yourself, when the children are grown up, when you have paid off the mortgage, etc.

Use the time to prepare for what you really care about – take classes, read books, get a few qualifications under your belt. That will make the whole transition period much easier.

But before you give up the idea of a new life, do look at the alternatives very carefully. Moving to a mountain-top instead of a crowded city can be running away, or you can organize it so that you become self-sufficient in most things, and perhaps make or grow something marketable which will turn into a respectably-profitable business.

The people around you
Sometimes you may feel it's not the job, but the people you work for and with that are upsetting you. If so, try and talk it over with the personnel manager or a friend who knows the situation. Or just consider whether it's your attitude that causes the difficulties. If not, if you genuinely feel that you are doing your best, then look around and see if you can find somewhere else, in the same sort of work.

When unemployment is high and especially in a limited job market, that may not be so easy. The only real help is to recognize that at present there's nothing you can do, and get interested in something outside of work, in a hobby or a sport, so the pinpricks at work don't bother you as much.

And if you don't trust someone, try to understand why you feel the way you do, get it out in the open and ask for an explanation. If that isn't satisfactory, break up any financial arrangement.

You don't know what you want
For youngsters this may not be so much of a problem. The ideal is to try as many different things as possible, so that you get a better idea of what is available. That doesn't mean two weeks here and two weeks there, either – you'll barely get to know your way around. But six months or so on a steady job should be enough to tell you if it's for you.

For older people professional help is probably more important. Try to find some sort of career counselling service, talk to a few agencies, get in touch with old friends in other fields. If you remember what interested you most at school, take a few courses at evening class, and see if it still makes you want to work in the same field.

And don't try to convince your children to settle down in something *they* don't like. That's the time to keep options open and it's the only time in their lives when they are not so likely to have many responsibilities.

Women and Work

Working women still face very special and conflicting emotions when it comes to working outside the home. Despite the women's movement, many people still believe that a woman's first responsibility is to her home and family, while work is a man's first care. The ideal solution is that both partners recognize that work-life and home-life should be of equal importance to you both – really imperative for a happy integrated life.

Husbands can be secretly of openly resentful about 'being neglected' and make their wives feel guilty about choosing to work. At work, a woman who is ambitious and career-minded still has quite a few hurdles to get over, as she seems to be a threat to nice, tidy sex groupings of secretaries and clerks in one lot, executives and professionals in another.

Often it is other women who resent the intruder most, and it can be occasionally very unpleasant. But it is important to keep a sense of proportion. More and more women are going out to work, and staying at work. Most of the obvious barriers are not really considered any more, and unusual jobs are opening up to both sexes.

A great many extra problems will come from your own attitude. If you are confident that you are serious about what you are doing, and take your job and your responsibilities as real challenges, then you'll have no time to worry about petty comments and snide remarks, and sooner or later they will just vanish as you all get on with getting the work done.

Job Identification

Most of us care deeply about the work that we do, but it shouldn't be allowed to become a substitute for self-confidence, or an ego-booster which gives us security because of our title. It may be pleasant enough while all is well, but if anything happens it may upset everything else in our lives. You may lose a job through ill health, through redundancy, through economic conditions, or just because you're not quite up to scratch. Finding another job may be difficult enough – to have to re-build a whole new set of convictions about yourself can seem overwhelmingly difficult. Too many suicides occur when people are fired – sometimes it's the refusal to face up to financial problems, but sometimes it is simply that being rejected at work has turned into being rejected as a human being. You are much more than your work, and never forget that for one moment.

MONEY AND YOU

Problems about money and household finances are all too common – money is a five-letter word, listed as being among the five top reasons for divorce. Yet the majority of the quarrels and complaints are not about how much money is coming in, but about how it is going out. Making a budget seems to be basic common sense, but all too often it's neglected until there is not a penny to pay the milkman but there's a new carpet in the dining room.

It is truly amazing how many couples get married when they have no idea about what they each consider important, what they would like to spend the income on, or even who is entitled to do the spending. Even today, many women don't even know what their husband earns, while other men turn over their pay packets dutifully and have no idea what will be bought or how it will be paid for. Both attitudes are way out of date.

Today's marriage should be a partnership, each one contributing money or services or both, each knowing they have agreed on the basic priorities, and each having something to spend as they please. If times are hard, there may not be much but at least it will be shared, and when things improve, then both will benefit, and the home will be something they have built together.

Children and money can be a problem, too. The amount of pocket money doesn't really matter, as long as it's around the same as most of the other children round about receive. Too much is just as bad as too little,

so don't be ashamed to ask other parents. They are usually only too happy for someone to take the initiative.

Make sure that you all understand what the pocket money is for. Set out as simply as possible whether you expect the child to buy only unnecessary things like chocolates and records or whether it includes clothes and school books. Helping a child to make up a budget is good training for both of you.

Money and Power
Too often having money seems to be confused with having power, and especially power over other people in or outside the family.

The excuse usually begins with wanting the best of everything for the ones you love, which is very understandable. But all too often, the excuse becomes the reason, and the *need* to have a great deal of money becomes an end in itself. Then if the supply is threatened, if failure looms on the horizon, the ego becomes terrified and panicky because money has become confused with self. If you believe that money is the basis for affection, then losing money will take love away. If you believe that money makes everybody around you respect you, then losing money must mean you lose their respect, and probably your self-respect, too. The snowballing effect of confusing yourself with your job or the money you earn can be hideously destructive.

Use money intelligently, use it carefully and for the benefit of everyone in the family on an equal basis. Then forget about it, if you can.

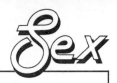
That sounds easy, but it isn't, in a world where other people may judge you by what you own. But they are the childish ones; remember that bits of paper and coins are tools – they should be useful and well-kept, but not worshipped. Use it to make what you want out of your life, don't let it use you.

A FAMILY BUDGET

Every family will have a different budget, but the main expenses are very similar. Put down your total income from all sources. Don't forget to make an allowance for income tax. Then add up what you need to spend every week, or every month, whichever is easier; rent or mortgage repayments, electricity and gas, telephones, necessary repairs, normal food bills, and so forth. Deduct these from your weekly or monthly income, and there should be something left over for

emergencies, and something to put aside to spend on family outings, special events, birthdays, etc. Don't forget about clothes – new shoes for all the children can totally upset a careful budget, and even shoe repairs can mount up terribly quickly.

If there is a little space between income and outgoings, then you should be all right. If not, then have another look at your spending budget, and see where you can cut down. Learning to make your own clothes can save quite a bit, so can doing your own house repairs, growing your own fruit and vegetables. Stop smoking and drink less hard liquor and you'll almost certainly become fitter and healthier in the bargain.

In other words, use your budget to get the best out of life instead of thinking of it as hardship or stinginess. Living the good life *can* be cheaper!

SEX AND SEXUAL RELATIONSHIPS

The problems that arise from human relationships are infinite; we are social animals, and if we become isolated from other human beings the damage to the human personality is frightening. We become withdrawn, first neurotic, and then totally unable to cope with the simplest requirements.

Living together also brings a certain amount of stress – we've seen some of the problems that may arise in the family. There are other

circumstances which create obvious conflicts – work, social conditions, even national divisions when politicians squabble, and countries quarrel over words in a treaty or boundary lines on a map.

For the ordinary person, though, the one special area likely to cause the most personal difficulties is sex and sexual relationships.

Perhaps this is the natural outcome of the fact that sex matters to us in one way or another for most of our lives. It is part of being a male or a female child, part of our earliest experiences as we discover the difference, and it may even affect our choice of career, and where we choose to live. As we grow older, a stable and loving sexual commitment is the best framework for a contented family life, and when all the responsibilities of children and work begin to fade away, we still find ourselves needing that closeness and companionship even more than ever before.

So it's not surprising that sex is considered the most powerful way of relating to each other, providing the deepest and greatest joy in our lives, but also unhappily the source of some of the greatest problems of adjustment and communication.

Many of the worst conflicts come from inside ourselves, and they are often based on ignorance. There has been more nonsense written and spoken about sex than about any other known subject. Some of the silliest myths have been around for years, perpetuating misery and unhappiness generation after generation, as we 'warn' our children or hide our fears from our parents.

Sex and love are inseparable
It is easy to recognize that the profoundest experience of sex is when it is linked to deep and abiding love, but they also exist quite separately, and have the right to be considered as individual ways of expressing emotion and sharing pleasure. After all, we accept that there are many kinds of love which are non-sexual – friends, teachers, religious leaders and fellow human beings may all share something of their experience

and much of their humanity with us.

Sex, too, has its own place in our daily lives, and it can be used – or abused. What matters most is that whatever form of satisfaction we choose should be mutually beneficial; caring about your partner's needs as well as your own is a basic human concern in even the briefest relationship.

Technique is all that matters
Once you know the mechanics, you will turn instantly into the greatest lover since Valentino. Not so! Sex is an art as well as a craft, and technique is only the beginning, the tool that you use to show tenderness and affection. Of course the more you know about the basic facts, the better you'll be able to understand what is happening to both of you. By all means read a good book, but remember that is the starting post, not the finishing line.

Men only want sex, women only want love
This particular myth is probably the most destructive of all, because it takes one of the basic human needs away from an entire sex.

We should begin to understand by now that a woman has sexual desires which can match or sometimes exceed her partner's. As we learn to cope with two grown-up sexes instead of one, girls are finally being allowed to have sexual feelings and responses which are an important part of every personality. The equivalent adjustment is not so obvious but is just as important – men need love and affection just as much as women do. When this need is repressed or pushed away because it isn't 'manly' then we only distort and diminish the human relationship.

Many men go through their lives refusing to admit that they even have emotions, let alone need to express them. Boys don't cry, soldiers aren't frightened, and fighting your way to the top is a ruthless claw-and-tooth struggle. But boys do cry, as any mother knows, the bravest soldier may scream in fear, and many successful businessmen would willingly hold out a hand to help a friend.

And this is just as true in a sexual relationship; once a man and woman realize that it really *is* a partnership, that men need to be held as well as to hold, and love as well as be loved, then much of the loneliness and pain which comes from isolation in a hard and frightening world will vanish.

Finally, one of the most common myths of all, *performance*; manhood is always potent, womenhood always means having an orgasm. Both false beliefs cause untold shame, embarrassment and guilt which can ruin even the warmest relationship.

To begin with, sex is a state of mind as well as a physical response. When a man is tired, worried, unhappy or disturbed his ability to function sexually is usually affected. Too much work and especially too much alcohol will smother sexual responses all too easily, and the simple answer is not in another woman, but in a little less work and a lot less alcohol.

Tired from a harrassing day with demanding young children, a woman may find it difficult to re-establish herself as an adult, and her lukewarm or even faked reaction is enough to discourage both partners from trying again. She feels guilty and wonders if she is frigid, he feels ashamed that he cannot make her happy, and unless they have enough sense to realize that both conditions created a temporary unimportant incident, it will happen over and over again, and it becomes self-perpetuating misery.

The answer is simple in principle, though sometimes difficult in practice – sex should be accepted as an open and wonderful part of your life, approached with a mixture of information and affection, a strong force in a sound and satisfying relationship. When problems occur, they should be treated with the same awareness and lack of shame we use to talk about other conflicts in our daily lives.

Human concern, respect for each other, responsibility, and just as important, a sharing of laughter and fun as well as joy – these should all be present, so that sex can be a source of happiness and strength for both of you.

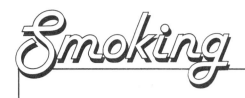

THE WORST ENEMY

You've heard it all before – in fact, you're fed up with hearing about it. You *know* cigarettes can cause cancer, but you also know of at least two or three pack-a-day people who coughed and wheezed a bit, but managed to survive to a reasonable age.

But, the fact is, cancer is not the only problem smoking cigarettes can cause. Smoking doesn't just kill you, it can also spoil your quality of life. For a start, it affects your everyday health. In addition to making you more prone to lingering colds, cigarettes actually use up an incredible amount of some of the vital vitamins. According to recent research, one cigarette destroys 25 mg. of vitamin C. They have the same affect on a group of substances called Lecithin, which work to keep fats moving through the bloodstream and stop cholesterol from forming.

And if this is not enough, there are horrifying statistics to come. Smokers are twice as likely to die before middle-age as non-smokers. Two out of five die before the age of 65, compared to one out of five non-smokers. And smokers are 70 times more likely to get lung cancer. In other words the cancer threat is not only real, it is serious. Equally alarming is that fact that the carbon monoxide given off by cigarettes is 400 times higher than the level considered safe for industry.

When you smoke, you are not only harming yourself, but you are jeopardizing the health of others. For example, a child's chance of getting pneumonia or bronchitis in the first

year of life nearly doubles if both parents smoke. Even if only one parent smokes, the child's chances of this type of lung ailment are 50 % greater. Smoking during pregnancy is more likely to lead to the birth of lighter-weight babies; and some studies have shown that incidence of crib death among babies born to smoking mothers is greater.

Your sex life can also be affected by smoking. According to recent research, over a period of years smoking actually begins to affect a man's ability to reach climax. It has also been conjectured that smoking affects sex hormones, causing menopause to occur early in smoking women.

Smoking is hard on the skin, causing wrinkling around the eyes at an earlier age. It's hard on tooth enamel, staining it so severely that even the most careful regular brushing will eventually not be able to remove it.

At last, even smokers must admit that the smoking habit involves some unpleasant side-affects. The smell of stale smokes permeates clothing and the air in a room to an unpleasant degree. It is disturbing to nonsmokers (and even some smokers) when people puff away in enclosed public places such as trains, airplanes, and buses. Even certain open areas such as restaurants are made unpleasant by smoking.

So why don't people just *stop*! The fact is, quitting smoking is not that easy, particularly for those people who are addicted. Nicotine is a *drug*, falling into the stimulant group. Like drinking, people often begin smoking because it is socially acceptable. Then due to the kick they get from the nicotine, the social smoking turns into a habit and the habit, combined with the drug becomes an addiction.

To stop smoking means to go through both the breaking of a habit and the withdrawing (albeit less severe than an alcohol or a hard drug withdrawal) from a drug. We all know how hard it is to break a habit, but when this is combined with extreme anxiety, jumpiness, depression, fatigue and a number of other physical symptoms that may accompany the withdrawal, it becomes extremely difficult.

But stopping is not impossible. Groups have been formed to aid people in kicking the smoking habit and they report a high degree of success. People have also been successful by just stopping cold. Not everyone becomes addicted to nicotine, and many of those who have stopped quickly or only smoke occasionally may well be among that group. Other aids and books have also come out on the market to help those who wish to stop.

Many people begin smoking – and continue smoking – in order to deal with daily stress. In fact, nicotine, like any other drug, has the paradoxical effect of starting off by making one feel less stressed, while, in fact, contributing greatly to overall anxiety – both physical and emotional.

There is no reason to smoke and there are a multitude of reasons to quit. Do it ... now!

SMOKING AND DISEASE

These are the diseases which we know show much higher death rates for smokers than for non-smokers:
Cancer of the lung, Cancer of the mouth, Cancer of the larynx, Cancer of the esophagus, Cancer of the prostate, Cancer of the pancreas, Coronary heart disease, Atheroscleosis and Thrombosis, Emphysema, Cirrhosis of the liver and Ulcers.

Pregnancy problems
A mother who is smoking during pregnancy is more likely to have a smaller, weaker baby who is already addicted to nicotine before it is born.

Senses
Smoking reduces the keeness of the sense of taste and the sense of smell. This may be part of the reason why sexual feelings may be reduced, and potency affected.

Pipe Smoking
Pipe tobacco probably contains more nicotine per ounce than most cigarette tobacco, but it burns at a much lower rate, and it is the temperature of burning which causes the carcogenins to form.

The ritual of filling a pipe, tamping down the tobacco, getting it to light, all cuts actual smoking time to a minimum. Chewing on an unlit pipe seems to satisfy many pipesmokers almost as much as smoking itself.

Too Much To Drink

ALCOHOLISM

Alcohol, more than any other drug, is used to ease everyday tensions; it is extremely potent, affecting the way we think, feel, and act. The effect of alcohol helps us to relax after a hard day of work and allows us to be more at ease socially. We drink to enhance appetite, to reduce appetite, to give energy, to help us sleep, to perk us up. In other words, it is used to alter our moods.

Because drinking is an activity that is not only condoned in our society, but looked upon by some as an expression of masculinity, and by others as one of the finer delights of life (even drunkeness is often considered amusing), it is very easy for anyone to slip from social drinking to alcohol addiction.

Why some people become alcoholics and others do not is unknown. Many psychologists believe that alcoholism is merely a sympton for severe psychological conflicts, beginning, in most cases, in early childhood. If a person with such chronic inner tensions turns to drink for relief, the chances of his becoming addicted are perhaps greater. Other experts feel that alcoholics suffer from a physical intolerance which is probably hereditary. The real answer may be a combination of the two elements.

The road into alcoholism is a predictible one, varying only in time. Some people become alcoholics quickly; for others, it may take years. Still others do not show a dependency on alcohol early in life, but as their active, productive years end, they turn to drinking to ease their tensions.

In the beginning, the alcoholic receives immense, perhaps profound, gratifiction from drink. Almost immediately he begins turning to it time and time again, each time searching for – and finding – tremendous relief. Sooner or later he develops a psychic dependence on alcohol, and then without knowing it, a physical one. Once the physical dependence exists, he will need to keep increasing his drinking to produce the same affect. Ultimately, he will suffer social, marital, emotional, physical, economic, and vocational complications, and in many cases, will die young, either by illness or accident. The hallmark of alcoholism is loss of control. The alcoholic is unable to control his behavior, not only his drinking behavior, but often his behavior in every other area of his life. He will drink more than he wants to or when he has promised himself to abstain. He finds himself lying to cover up either his drinking or the results of his drinking. Moreover, the disease is characterized by an inability to be objective and to face reality. Once the addiction has taken hold, the last reality the alcoholic wants to face is that he is addicted and must give up alcohol. He must have a drink at all costs, and he will sacrifice anything to get it.

Alcoholism used to be thought of as a 'moral' problem, treatable only through religious instruction and the Salvation Army. Today, people are far more realistic. They recognize that alcoholism is a disease and must be treated as such. However, like most diseases, it must be treated by experts. Some general practitioners are ill-equipped to treat the alcoholic and frequently concentrate on the physical symptoms such as cirrhosis of the liver instead of the addiction and its cures. In fact, well-intentioned doctors have occasionally held an alcoholic's hand right to the grave.

If you suspect that you or a member of your family might be addicted to alcohol, see your doctor and talk frankly as soon as possible. Find out if, in fact, alcoholism is the problem. If so, investigate the most effective method of cure. Alcoholics Anonymous is the most famous and most effective organization. There are A.A. offices in every major city in Britain and the United States. Also, most major hospitals have alcoholism units and are excellent sources of advice. Whatever you do, get help.

Antabuse

Antabuse is the trade name for the chemical compound, disulfirma and is often used to help abstaining alcoholics *not* take that one fatal drink. Alone, it has no effect, but when taken with alcohol, it interferes with the way the body absorbs the drink. Through a complicated chemical reaction, Antabuse produces increased blood pressure which results in flushing of the face, pounding in the temples, and accelerated heartbeat. Headache often develops and frequently a difficulty in breathing is noticed which may, in turn, result in coughing. Finally, there is often an emotional reaction characterized by extreme anxiety. In other words, if you take an Antabuse tablet and later (within 3 days) take a drink, you will become very sick! Antabuse is best used by alcoholics who are highly motivated to stop drinking, but find that despite all their efforts, they maintain a profound craving for alcohol. Patients must

always be tested for Antabuse use because each person's response varies. Also Antabuse should never be given surreptitiously. Despite these restrictions and warnings, the use of Antabuse among certain alcoholic patients has been highly successful. It is an aid well worth considering.

15 SYMPTOMS OF POSSIBLE ALCOHOLISM

1. A preoccupation with drinking
2. Drinking in the morning, or at any other inappropriate time
3. A need to drink to perform adequately at work or socially
4. Feeling, in general, that drinking is a necessity
5. Guilt over the necessity to drink
6. Experience with alcohol amnesias or blackouts
7. Drop in work efficiency and professional absenteeism
8. Comments from an employer, relatives, or friends
9. Deterioration of human relationships linked to drinking
10. Justification for drinking with self-deception
11. Reduction in sexual drive
12. Concealing liquor and/or sneaking drinks
13. Repeated attempts to stop drinking which fail
14. Neglect of meals in order to drink
15. Physical and mental symptoms such as cirrhosis of the liver, peripheral neuritis, psychiatric complication, delirium tremens, and other drink-related diseases.

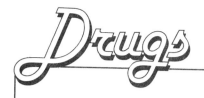

OTHER DRUG PROBLEMS

Drug abuse might be defined as an inability to control the use of a drug. The result is that the addict harms himself, members of the family, and other members of society.

The use of drugs to escape the drudgery or pain of life has been a part of society through history. In recent years, to a great degree because the middle class parents have suddenly been faced with their youngsters becoming heroin addicts or being arrested for possessing marijuana, drug abuse has seemingly become a bigger and bigger problem. The fact is that the problem, in one form or another, has always been with us.

Types of drugs
The most serious drugs are the *opium derivative* drugs including *morphine, codeine,* and *heroin*. Once an addiction to any of these drugs has been established, the victim's entire emotional life is subjugated to the need to find adequate supplies.

Habit-forming drugs cause two kinds of problems. Once dependent, the addict feels a need to continue his dependence due to a profound craving; this is reinforced by the feeling of extreme elation he feels once he has taken the drug.

Heroin is perhaps the The import of heroin into most countries is illegal, so it must be smuggled in, making the cost of buying it prohibitive. Unless the addict is on a registered addiction, he must turn to crime.

Withdrawal from heroin is characterized by acute physical pain – severe cramps in the abdomen and legs, muscular twitching, and diarrhoea. The patient will be totally unable to relax, rest, or sleep. Treatment for withdrawal should be conducted only by well-trained experts and psychotherapy is almost always required.

Cocaine is a drug which in recent years has attained a certain popularity among chic, upper class young adults as well as people in the entertainment fields. Cocaine is taken by sniffing through the nostrils and it produces a feeling of elation. Sometimes, however, cocaine can produce hallucinations and even psychosis. An overdose can result in death.

*Hallucinogens,*the most common being marijuana and LSD, are a group of drugs that produce an euphoric effect. Marijuana is made from dried leaves of Indian hemp which grows wild throughout the world. Hashish is another by-product of hemp and can be 5 to 10 times as potent as marijuana. Marijuana and hashish are usually rolled in cigarettes and smoked, although they can be also be cooked in foods such as 'brownies'. It has many nicknames – pot, grass, reefers, joints, tea – and produces a sensation of floating, a gross distortion of time and space, and a feeling of relaxation and euphoria which lasts for a few hours. Marijuana is not addictive, although there is some evidence that long-term use can cause chromosomal changes resulting in birth defects in future generations.

LSD is an hallucinogenic drug derived from a fungus and produces vivid images, combining visual, auditory, tactile, and olfactory sensations that are pleasurable to some and terrifying to others. In the 1960s, LSD received a tremendous amount of publicity glorifying its mind-expanding properties, but most people now accept it as not only useless, but producing negative effects. While it is not known to be addictive, instances of 'bad trips', some resulting in death, have been numerous. It has also been reported that hallucinations can recur weeks or months after taking the drug.

The youth cult of the sixties instigated more public interest in drug addiction, but, in fact, dependence on drugs has existed among middle class adults for centuries – many times without the person being aware that he is a drug addict.

Drugs commonly used to ease everyday tensions include the *bromides,* the *barbiturates, and the stimulants.*

Bromides are sedatives made from compounds of bromine and are often used for hangovers. Bromides are not addictive, but they can have a negative cumulative affect on the system. Bromide intoxication, or an excess of bromide in the blood, causes drowsiness, delirium, hallucination, and occasionally, death. Hospitalization is usually required.

Barbiturates are made from an organic compound or barituric acid. They make the taker feel relaxed and are often used as sleeping aids and also to relieve tension during periods of distress. The popular sedatives, Valium and Librium fall into this group. Barbiturates can become addictive, and like alcohol, require greater and greater dosages to achieve the desired affect. Withdrawal from barbiturates is characterized by increased anxiety which often prompts the addict to take even more. Treatment for barbiturate addiction is difficult and may require hospitalization.

Stimulants are still another group of commonly-used drugs. The most popular and most frequently used is caffeine which is found in coffee, tea, cocoa, and cola beans. (Little comment is needed on how much coffee is consumed in the United States, tea in Britain, and chocolate in both countries.) Contrary to common belief, very little of the stimulant from the cola bean is found in any of the commercial cola drinks.

Other *stimulants* include the *amphetamines* (*benzedrine, dexedrine* and *methedrine.*) Amphetamines are taken as 'uppers' or 'pep pills', stimulate drive and can create an overall feeling of happiness. They are often used as diet pills because they depress the appetite, and also for relief of depression. 'Speed' is the slang term for amphetamines. Some people dissolve the pills in liquid and then shoot the drug directly into the veins. Done in excess over a long period of time, this kind of 'mainlining' as it is called, can be lethal.

Addiction is a very serious problem, difficult to identify and painful to cure. But like alcoholism, it does not carry the moral stigma it once did, and if you suspect that either you or a member of your family may be addicted, don't be ashamed – get help immediately.

PSYCHOANALYSIS

Some of us come to the point where coping with the normal stresses of everyday life are so overwhelming that living from day to day — and often from crisis to crisis — is extremely painful. If we have tried to discuss our problems with relatives and friends or to escape on a vacation or into a hobby, but nothing seems to work, psychoanalysis may well be a healthy alternative.

Psychoanalysis, for years, bore the stigma of being a solution open to only those who were considered truly crazy. This stigma no longer holds true. Modern philosophers and many average citizens believe that most of us are neurotic in some way, and if our neuroses begin to intrude on the productive functioning of our lives, psychoanalysis can be a positive and useful remedy.

By definition, psychoanalysis is a method of determining patterns of emotional thinking and development. Based on the analytical techniques originated by Sigmund Freud, psychoanalysis uses free association of thoughts, dream interpretation, and an analyses of resistance and transference to reveal to the conscious mind various thoughts, feelings and ways of behaving that were previously unconscious. The theory is that emotions that were once painful were repressed, but nevertheless, left an imprint on the mind that lead to exaggerated emotional responses or distorted thinking and behavior. When these thoughts are made conscious, the patient is then free to deal with them. Of course, many problems that are discussed in therapy are conscious ones. Together with the therapist, the patient seeks ways to make maximum use of his resources, modify stressful conditions in his environment, and change negative patterns of behavior. Psychoanalysis therapy is done over a period of time (the amount of time depends on how complex or deep-seated the problems are) through extensive interviews between two people, the patient and a therapist, who is either a psychiatrist or a psychologist. A psychiatrist is a licensed physician, specially trained to practice psychoanalysis. A psychologist is a doctor (PhD) of psychology and in most places must be certified to practice. A psychiatrist, being a medical doctor, can prescribe drugs (which can include anything from mild tranquilizers to potent anti-psychotic pills) or administer other medical techniques. A psychologist cannot prescribe drugs.

Types of Therapy

Many types of therapy are available. With regard to so-called 'classical' therapy, the question is frequently asked 'Is the therapist a Freudian therapist?' The answer is that *all* psychiatrists and psychologists are Freudian in the sense that Freud originated the concepts that are the standard frame of reference.

But any licensed therapist has also studied the psychoanalytic theories of many other pioneers in the field (Jung, Rank, and Horney, to name a few) and most have incorporated these people's methods into their own way of functioning. Rather than worry about what kind of therapist a doctor is, it is far better to see if a constructive relationship can be cultivated between the two of you. Only through trust can constructive therapy result.

Group Therapy

In group therapy, a number of patients (usually about six or eight) meet together to discuss their problems. A professional therapist is always present to moderate the session.

Group therapy can be particularly useful if you have considerable problems dealing with other people. If you are overly shy, you will be forced, in a sense, to communicate and will usually receive the support of others in the group. If you are overly aggressive, arrogant, or sadistic, these trends will also be pointed out by the others and the therapist.

Group therapy can also be a supportive environment for most everyday problems. Such groups tend to give one helpful suggestions for coping with problems, and you quickly learn that you are not alone.

Marital Therapy

There are infinite ways to conduct therapy for troubled married couples, and any creative therapist will work with couples to find a way that will be successful. One method is to use two therapists (often it is helpful to have one therapist be male and the other female) together with the couple. This way, both partners can be observed by both therapists, ideas have fertile ground for analysis, and usually the threat of one partner feeling that he or she is 'teacher's pet' is lessened if not obliterated.

Marital therapy can be tremendously useful. Airing problems that one simply cannot communicate in a one-to-one situation is made easier. Your ways of dealing with each other are analyzed, frequently pointing out types of behavior that might never have been noticed by either partner, but were having a detrimental affect on the relationship.

Sex therapy is one kind of marital therapy. Masters and Johnson are pioneers in this field, but many hospitals and clinics have adopted either their techniques or similar ones. The objective is basic – to help couples communicate their needs, specifically their sexual needs, in a constructive and sympathetic situation. The inability to relate sexually is one of the greatest causes of divorce, but sex therapy has proved to have a high success rate.

Rehabilitation Therapy

Many social problems including alcoholism, drug addiction, and various criminal offences, are considered by psychologists to be merely symptoms of severe psychiatric difficulties. Once the illness (in the case of addiction) or the offence has been treated, it is important to seek psychiatric help to make sure the patient does not return to addiction or crime.

Above all, remember that psychoanalysis as counselling is no longer considered taboo. Today we believe that mental illnesses deserve the same amount of empathy and attention that physical diseases merit. After all, if you suspected you had a cancerous growth, you would be tested immediately and have it treated. The same holds true for unhealthy emotions. It is important to have any kind of suspected sickness treated quickly and with understanding.

Appendix

Useful References

DIET & NUTRITION

Weight Control Dynamics Ltd.
171 West 57th Street
New York, New York 10019

Weight Control Specialists
176 East 75th Street
New York, New York 10021

Weight & Smoking Control Information Center
36 East Broadway
New York, New York 10003
212–226–6036

Weight Watchers' Incorporated
111 Broadway
New York, New York 10036
212–962–7760

Weight Watchers' Camps Incorporated
138 Madison Avenue
New York, New York 10016
212–889–9500

Weight Watchers' International
800 Community Drive
Manhasset, Long Island, New York
516–627–9200

Weight Watchers' Magazine
635 Madison Avenue
New York, New York 10022
212–838–8964

Nutrition Center
247 East 50th Street
New York, New York 10021
212–753–5363

Nutrition & Diet Tips
93 Worth Street
New York, New York 10003
212–431–4540

Nutrition Foundation Inc.
589 Fifth Avenue
New York, New York 212–687
212–687–4830

Nutrition Institute of America
200 West 86th Street
New York, New York 10036
212–595–7507

ALCOHOLISM

Alcohol Abuse & Alcoholism
Intervention Center
Louden Avenue
Amityville, New York
516–264–5001

SMOKING

SmokEnders: The Jacquelyn Rogers Method
145 East 52nd Street
New York, New York 10022
212–751–6060

NUTRITION

Chaney, Margaret S. & Ross, Margaret L., *Nutrition*. Boston: Houghton-Mifflin, 1971

Darden, Ellington, *Nutrition for Athletes*. New York: Anna Publications, 1975

Dinaberg, Kathy & Akel, D'An, *Nutrition Survival Kit: A Wholefoods Recipe & Reference Guide*. San Francisco: Panjandrum Press, 1976

Emily Post Institute, *Nutrition for Your Family's Health*. New York: Essandess, 1970

Gifft, Helen, et.al., *Nutrition, Behavior & Change*. Englewood Cliffs: Prentice-Hall, 1972

Jacobson, Michael F., *Nutrition Scoreboard*. New York: Avon Books, 1975

Katch, Frank I., & McArdle, William D., *Nutrition, Weight Control & Exercise*. Boston: Houghton-Mifflin, 1977

Kirschman, J. D., *Nutrition Almanac*. New York: McGraw-Hill, Yearly publication

Kreitzman, Stephen & Kreitzman, Susan, *Nutrition Cookbook: 123 Gourmet Recipes Computer Analyzed for Your Specific Daily Requirements*. New York: Harcourt, Brace, Jovanovich, 1977

Moghissi, Kamran S., & Evans, Tommy N., *Nutrition Impacts on Women*. New York: Harper & Row, 1977

Morella, Joseph J, & Turchette, Richard J., *Nutrition & the Athlete*. New York: Mason Charter, 1975.

Pike, Ruth L, & Brown, Myrtle, L. *Nutrition: An Integrated Approach*. New York: John Wiley, 1975

Runyon, Thora J., *Nutrition for Today*. New York: Harper & Row, 1976

Stare, Frederick J. & McWilliams, Margaret, *Nutrition for Good Health*. New York: Plycon Press, 1974

Watson, George, *Nutrition & Your Mind*. New York: Bantam Books, 1974

Williams, Roger J., *Nutrition Against Disease*. New York: Bantam Books, 1974

Williams, Roger J., *Nutrition in a Nutshell*. New York: Doubleday, 1977

Winick, Myron (Ed.), *Nutrition & Aging*. New York: John Wiley, 1976

BASIC COOKBOOKS

Anderson, Jean & Hanna, Elaine, *The Doubleday Cookbook*. New York: Doubleday, 1976

Anderson, Jean, *The Family Circle Cookbook*. New York: Simon & Schuster, 1976

Beard, James, *American Cookery*. New York: Knopf, 1976

Becker, Irma Rombauer, *The Joy of Cooking*. New York: Bobbs-Merrill, 1976 (Latest edition)

Child, Julia & Beck, Simone, *Mastering the Art of French Cooking*. (Volumes I & II) New York: Knopf, 1965

Farmer, Fannie, *The Fannie Farmer Cookbook*. Boston: Little Brown, 1976 (latest edition)

Hewitt, Jean & Staff, *The American Heritage Cookbook*. New York: Bantam Books, 1976

Seranne, Ann, *Ann Seranne's Good Food & How to Cook It*. New York: William Morrow & Company, 1972

DIETING

Bond, Clara-Beth Y., *Low Fat, Low Cholesterol Diet*. New York: Doubleday, 1977

Bruno, Frank J., *Think Yourself Thin: How Psychology Can Help You Lose Weight*. New York: Barnes & Noble, 1975

Casale, Joan T., *Diet Food Finer*. New York: R. R. Bowker, 1975

Cheraskin, E., *Diet & Disease*. Scranton: Rodale, 1968

Cole, William & Perlstein, Irving B., *Diet is Not Enough*. New York: MacMillan, 1968

Fiore, Evelyn L., *Low Carbohydrate Diet*. New York: Grossett & Dunlap, 1965

Fredericka, Carlton, & Goodman, Herman, *Low Blood Sugar & You*. New York: Grossett & Dunlap, 1969

Goldbeck, Nikki & Goldbeck, David, *Dieter's Companion: A Guide to Nutritional Self-Sufficiency*. New York: McGraw-Hill, 1975

Hittleman, Richard, *Weight Control Through Yoga*. New York: Bantam Books, 1974

Hurdle, J. Frank, *Low Blood Sugar: A Doctor's Guide to Its Effective Control*. Englewood Cliffs: Prentice-Hall, 1969

Jones, Jeanne, *Diet for a Happy Heart*. San Francisco: One-Hundred-One Productions, 1975

Mayer, Jean, *Diet for Living*. New York: McKay, 1975

Milo, Mary, & Family Circle Staff, *Diet & Exercise Guide*. New York: Arno Books, 1976

Moore, Marci & Douglas, Mark, *Diet, Sex & Yoga*. New York: Arcane Books, 1970

Morrison, Lester M., *Low-Fat Way to Health & Longer Life*. New York: Arc Books, 1970

Palm, Daniel, *Diet Away Your Stress, Tension & Anxiety*. New York: Doubleday, 1976

Riccio, Dolores, & Riccio, Ottone, *The Weighing Game & How to Win It*. Scranton: Rodale Press, 1974

Runner's World Editors, *Runners' Diet*. New York: World, 1972

Schauf, Gworge E., *Think Thin*. New York: Fawcett, 1977

Small, Marvin, *Low-Calorie Diet.*, New York: Pocket Books, 1970

Smith, E. W., *Dietors Checklist*. New York: Doubleday, 1975

Wordsworth, Julie, *Diet Revolution*, New York: MacMillan, 1968

SPECIALTY COOKBOOKS

Black, Colette, *Low-Calorie Cookbook*. New York: MacMillan, 1962

Blevin, Marge & Ginder, Gerri, *Low-Blood Sugar Cookbook*. New York: Doubleday, 1973

Brownlee, Harriet, *The Low-Carbohydrate Gourmet: A Cookbook for Hungry Dieters*. New York: Morrow, 1975

Burros, Marian Fox, *Pure & Simple*. New York: William Morrow & Company, 1978

Caviani, Mable, *Low-Cholesterol Cookbook*. New York: Barnes & Noble, 1974

Dannet, Sylvia G. & McCabe, Maureen, *Low-Blood Sugar Gourmet Cookbook*. New York Barnes & Noble, 1975

Davis, Francyne, *Low-Blood Sugar Cookbook*. New York: Grosset & Dunlap, 1973

Gold, Ann, *Diet Watchers' Dessert Book*. New York: Grosset & Dunlap, 1974

Gold Ann & Briller, T., *Diet Watchers' Gourmet Cookbook*. New York: Grosset & Dunlap, 1975

Hecht, Nancy A., *Low-Cost Main Dishes*. New York: Arno Press, 1976

Lindeman, Joanne, *Low-Carbohydrate Cookbook*. San Francisco: Nitty Gritty, 1974

Marsh, Ann, *Beauty Recipes from Natural Foods*. New York: Stirling, 1974

Nidetch, Jean. *Weight Watcher's Program Cookbook*. New York: New American Library, 1977

Ross, Elain, *Low-Calorie Menus for Entertaining*. New York: Hastings House, 1970

Stead, Evelyn S. & Warren, Gloria K., *Low-Fat Cookery*. New York: McGraw-Hill, 1977

Sunset Editors, *Low-Cost Cookery*. Los Angeles: Sunset/Lane, 1976

Thorne, William, *Low-Carbohydrate Dieter's Cookbook*. New York: Pinnacle Books, 1973

Waldo, Myra, *Diet Delight Cookbook*. New York: MacMillan, 1977

FITNESS

Larson and Michelman, *International Guide to Fitness and Health*, Crown, 1973.

GENERAL ATHLETICS

Associations

Amateur Athletic Union of the United States
3400 West 86th Street
Indianapolis, Indiana 46268

Books

Boy Scouts of America, *Sports*. Indianapolis: Boy
Scouts of America, 1972

Casady, Donald R., *Sport Activities for Men*. New
York: MacMillan, 1974

Johnson, Perry B. *Sport Exercise and You*. New
York: Holt, Rinehart, & Winston. 1975

ARCHERY

Associations

American Archery Council
618 Chalmers Street
Flint, Michigan 48503

National Archery Association of the U.S.
1952 Geraldson Drive
Lancaster, Pennsylvania 17601

National Field Archery Association
Route 2, Box 514
Redlands, California

Books

Burke, Edmund, *Archery Handbook*. New York:
Arco Books, 1977

Gillelan, G. Howard, *The Complete Book of Bows
& Arrows*. Harrisburg: Stackpole, 1977

Heath, Ernest, G., *Better Archery*. London: Kaye &
Ward, 1977

BADMINTON

Associations

American Badminton Association
1330 Alexandria Drive
San Diego, California 92104

Books

Devein, Frank J. *Sports Illustrated Book of Badminton*. Philadelphia: Lippincot, 1973.

BALLET & DANCE

Books

Arnheim, Daniel & Schlaich, Joan, *Dance Injuries:
Their Prevention and Cure*. New York: Mosby,
1975

Featherstone, Donals F. & Allen, Rona, *Dancing
without Danger: The Prevention and Treatment
of Ballet Dancing Injuries*. New York: A. S.
Barnes, 1970

Le Maitre, Jerome & Chauvier, Yvette, *Dance for
Children*. New York; A. S. Barnes, 1977

White, Betty, *Dancing Made Easy*. New York:
Avon Books, 1976

    Dance Facilities. American Alliance for
Health Physical Education & Recreation, 1972

BALLROOM and COUNTRY DANCING

Books

Fallon, Dennis J. *The Art of Ballroom Dancing*.
Minneapolis: Burgess Publishing Company,
1977

Jensen and Jensen, *Square Dancing*, Brigham,
1973

BASEBALL

Associations

Amateur Softball Association of America
P.O. Box 11437
Oklahoma City, Oklahoma 73111

American Amateur Baseball Congress
212 Plaza Building
2855 West Market Street
Akron, Ohio 44131

National Amateur Baseball Federation
Route 1, Box 280B
Rose City, Missouri

Books

Editors of Sports Illustrated, *Sports Illustrated Book
of Baseball*. Philadelphia: Lippincott, 1972

BASKETBALL

Associations

American Basketball Association
1700 Broadway (42nd Floor)
New York, New York 10019

Books

Editors of Sports Illustrated, *The Sports Illustrated Book of Basketball*, Philadelphia: Lippincott, 1971

Schaafsma, Frances, *Basketball for Women*. Dubuque, Iowa W. C. Brown, 1977

BICYCLING

Associations

Amateur Bicycle League of America
P.O. Box 699
Wall Street Station,
New York, New York 10005

American Cycling Union
125 Carolina Avenue
Newark, New Jersey 07106

Books

Donner, Michael, *Bike, Skate & Skateboard Games*. New York: Golden Press, 1977

Dempsey, Paul, *The Bicyclers' Bible*. Summit, Pa.: Tab Books, 1977

George, Barbara, *Bicycle Road Racing*. Minneapolis: Lerner, 1977

George, Barbara, *Bicycle Track Racing*. Minneapolis: Lerner, 1977

Woodland, Les, *Cycle Racing & Touring*. London: Pelham, 1977

BODY BUILDING & WEIGHTLIFTING

Associations

America Weight Lifting Association
73 Main Street
Mechanicsburg, Pennsylvania

Books

Gaines, Charles, & Butler, George, *Pumping Iron*. New York: Simon & Schuster, 1975

Lance, Kathleen, *Getting Strong*, Bobbs Merrill, 1977

Kirkley, George W., *Weightlifting & Weight Training*. New York: Arco Books, 1966

Ryan, Frank, *Weight Training*. New York: The Viking Press, 1969

BOWLING

Associations

National Bowling Association
1806 Madison Avenue, Suite 407–408
Toledo, Ohio 43624

American Lawn Bowls Association
10337 Cheryl Drive
Sun City, Arizona 85351

Books

Anthony, Earl, *Winning Bowling*. Chicago: Contemporary Books, 1977

Sperber, Paula, *Inside Bowling for Women*. Chicago: Contemporary Books, 1977.

BOXING & WRESTLING

Associations

World Boxing Association
Mezzanine, Seelback Hotel
500 South 4th Street
Louisville, Kentucky 40202

U.S. Amateur Wrestling Foundation
c/o Powers Chemco
Charles Street
Glen Cove, New York 11542

Books

Wrestling. (Know the Game Series) New York: British Book Service, 1976

Sparks, Raymond E., *Wrestling Illustrated*. New York: Ronald Press, 1960

Thompson, Clayton, *Wrestling for Fun*. New York: A. S. Barnes, 1973

CANOEING & ROWING

Associations

American Canoe Association
4260 East Evans Avenue
Denver, Colorado 80222

American Rowing Association
4 East River Drive
Fairmount Park
Philadelphia, Pennsylvania 19130

Books

Bridge, Raymond, *Complete Guide to Kayaking*. New York: Scribners, 1977

Rude, W., *Canoeing and Kayaking*, McGraw Hill, 1974

CHILDREN'S GAMES

Books

Ford, Phyllis, *Informal Recreational Activities: A Leaders' Guide*. Martinsville: American Camping Association. 1977

Kramer, Jack, *Backyard Games: A Handbook for Homeowners & Gardeners*. New York: Berkeley, 1977

Krause, Richard G., *Recreation Today*. Santa Monica: Goodyear Publishing Co., 1977

Leverich, Kathleen, *Cricket's Expedition: Indoor & Outdoor Activities*. New York: Random House, 1977

CLIMBING

Associations

Adirondack Mountain Club
172 Ridge Street
Glen Falls, New York 12801

Appalachian Mountain Club
5 Joy Street
Boston, Massachusetts 02108

Books

Calder, Jean. *Walking: A Guide to Beautiful Walks & Trails*. New York: William Morrow & Company, Inc., 1977

Krochmal, Arnold & Krochmal, Connie, *Walker's Guide to Nature*. New York: Drake, 1977

Unger, Len, Walking: *The Perfect Exercise*. Impact Publications, 1976

Zochert, Donald, *Walking in America*. New York: Knopf, 1974

CURLING

Associations

U.S. Men's Curling Association
119 Monona Avenue
Madison, Wisconsin 53702

U.S. Women's Curling Association
1420 Clifton Park Road
Schenectady, New York 12308

Books

Mulvoy, Mark & Richardson, Ernie, *The Sports Illustrated Book of Curling*. Philadelphia: Lippincott, 1973

FENCING

Associations

Amateur Fencers League of America
249 Eton Place
Westfield, New Jersey 07090

Books

Lownds, Camille, *Foil Around & Stay Fit: Exercise Secrets of a Fencer*. New York: Harcourt, Brace, Jovanovich, 1977

FOOTBALL

Books

Wilkinson, Bud & Eds. *The Sports Illustrated Book of Football: Defense*, 1973. Philadelphia: Lippincott, 1973

Wilkinson, Bud & Eds. *The Sports Illustrated Book of Football: Offense*. Philadelphia: Lippincott, 1972

Wilkinson, Bud & Eds. *The Sports Illustrated Book of Football: Quarterback*. Philadelphia: Lippincott, 1972

GOLF

Associations

U.S. Golf Assocation
Golf House
Far Hills, New Jersey 07931

Books

Price, Charles & Editors, *The Sports Illustrated Book of Golf:* Philadelphia: Lippincott, 1972

HOCKEY

Associations

Field Hockey Association of America
1160 3rd Avenue
New York, New York 10021

U.S. Field Hockey Association
107 School House Lane
Philadelphia, Pennsylvania 19144

Amateur Hockey Association of the U.S. (Ice Hockey)
10 Lake Circle
Colorado Springs, Colorado 80906

Books

Staff of Sports Illustrated, *The Sports Illustrated Book of Ice Hockey*. Philadelphia: Lippincott, 1973

RUNNING & JOGGING

Associations

National Jogging Association
1910 K Street NW (Suite 202)
Washington, D.C. 20006

Road Runners
P.O. Box 112
Northbrook, Illinois 60062

Books

Dunaway, James O. and Staff of Sports Illustrated, *The Sports Illustrated Book of Track, Field, and Running Events*. Philadelphia: Lippincott, 1971

Fixx, James, *The Complete Book of Running*. New York: Random House, 1977.

Henderson, Joe & Eds., *Running with Style*. New York: World Publishers, 1975.

Lance, Kathryn, *Running for Health & Beauty*. New York: Bobbs-Merrill, 1977.

Runners' World Editors, *Runners; Training Guide*. New York: World Publishers, 1973

Runners' World Editors, *Running After Forty*. New York: World Publishers, 1975

Runners' World Editors, *Runners' Body*. New York: World Publishers. 1973

Spino, Mike, *Running Home: The Body & Mind Family Fitness Book*. San Francisco: Celestial Arts, 1977

THE MARTIAL ARTS

Associations

U.S. Judo Federation
R.R. 21 Box 519
Terre Haute, Indiana 47802

United Karate Federation
315 7th Avenue
New York, New York 10001

Books

Dominy, Eric, *Karate: Self-Taught*. New York: Bobbs-Merrill, 1976

Russell, W. Scott, *Karate: The Energy Connection*. New York: Delacorte, 1976

Schroeder, Charles R. & Wallace, Bill, *Karate: Basic Concepts & Skills*. New York: A & W Books, 1976

Tegner, Bruce, *Karate & Judo: Exercises for the Oriental Sport-Fighting Arts*. San Francisco: Thor, 1972

Tenjawarn, S., *Thai Boxing*. New York: Wehman, 1971

RIDING

Associations

American Horse Shows Association
527 Madison Avenue
New York
N.Y., USA

U.S. Pony Clubs
303 South High Street
West Chester
Pennsysvania 19380
U.S.A.

Books

Clayton, Michael and Steinkraus, William C., *The Complete Book of Show Jumping*, Crown, New York, 1977

Crago, Judy, *Junior Show Jumping*, T.Y. Crowell, 1977

RUGBY

Associations

Eastern Rugby Union of America
27 East State Street
Sherburn, New York 13460

Books

Rugby League Football (Know the Game Series). New York: British Book Service, 1976.

Creek, F. N. & Rutherford, Don, *Rugby*. (Teach Yourself Series) New York: McKay, 1975

Williams, Ray. *Rugby for Beginners*. New York: Souvenir International School Book Series, 1977.

SKATING

Associations

Society of Roller Skating Teachers of America
7700 A Street
Lincoln, Nebraska 68510

Books

Deegan, Paul J., *Skates & Skating*. New York: Watts, 1976

Scott, Barbara A., & Kirby, Michael, *Skating for Beginners*. New York: Knopf, 1976

SKATEBOARDING

Books

Cassorla, Albert, *Skateboarder's Bible*. San Francisco: Running Press, 1976

Grant, Jack, *Skateboarding: A Complete Guide to the Sport*. San Francisco: Celestial Arts, 1976

Weir, LaVada, *Skateboards & Skate Boarding: The Complete Beginners, Guide*. San Francisco: Missner, 1977

SKIING

Associations

U.S. Ski Association
1726 Champa Street (Suite 300)
Denver, Colorado 80202

Books

Skiing. (Know the Game Series) New York: British Book Center, 1976

Baldwin, Ned, *Skiing Cross Country*. New York: McGraw-Hill, 1977

Pfeiffer, Doug, *Skiing for Beginners*. New York: Atheneum, 1978

SOCCER

Associations

U.S. Soccer Football Association
Room 4010
350 Fifth Avenue
New York, New York 10001

Books

Beim, George, *Principles of Modern Soccer*. Boston;
Houghton-Mifflin, 1977

Marcus, Joe, *The Complete World of Soccer*. New
York: W. W. Norton, 1977

SQUASH & HANDBALL

Associations

U.S. Handball Association
4101 Dempster Street
Skokie, Illinois 60067

U.S. Squash Racquets Association
211 Ford Road
Bala-Cynwyd, Pennsylvania 19004

U.S. Women's Squash Racquets Association
Mustin Lane
Villanove, Pennsylvania 19085

Books

McFarland, Wayne J. & Philip Smith, *The Sports Illustrated Book of Handball*. Philadelphia: Lippincott, 1976

Staff of Sports Illustrated, *The Sports Illustrated
Book of Squash*. Philadelphia: Lippincott, 1971

SWIMMING, DIVING & OTHER WATER SPORTS

Associations

U.S. Swimming Association
P.O. Box 12184
Fresno, California 93776
Executive Director: Thomas O. Hiller

National Association of Underwater Instructors
22809 Barton Road
Grand Terrace, California 92324
General Manager: Arthur H. Ullrich, Jr.

Wester Surfing Association
4430 Alhambra Street
San Diego, California 92107
Executive Director: Judo Moser

Books

Athans, George, *Waterskiing*. New York: St. Mar-
tin's Press, 1975

Council for National Cooperation in Aquatics,
Swimming & Diving: A Bibliography. Association Press, 1969

Higgins, John F. et. al., *Swimming & Diving*. New
York: Arco Books, 1973

Staff of Sports Illustrated, *The Sports Illustrated
Book of Swimming & Diving*. Philadelphia: Lippincott, 1973

Staff of Sports Illustrated, *The Sports Illustrated
Book of Skin Diving & Snorkeling*, 1973

Walker, Morton, *Sport Diving: An Instructional
Guide to Skin and Scuba*. New York: Contempo
Books, 1977

TABLE TENNIS

Associations

U.S. Table Tennis Association
P.O. Box 815 EA
Orange, Connecticut 06477

Books

Miles, Dick, *The Sports Illustrated Book of Table
Tennis*. Philadelphia: Lippincott, 1974

LAWN TENNIS

Associations

U.S. Tennis Association
51 East 42nd Street
New York, New York 10017

National Baddleball Association
Sports Building
University of Michigan
Ann Arbor, Michigan 48104

Books

Cutler, Merritt M. *Tennis Book*. New York: McGraw-Hill, 1967

Hines, Henry & Morgenstern, Carol, *Quick Tennis: The Professional's Method for Quickness, Mobility, & Court Control — The Secret Ingredient in Winning Tennis*. New York: E. P. Dutton, 1977

Kraft, Steven, *Tennis Drills for Self-Improvement*. New York: Doubleday, 1978

Talbert, Bill, et. al., *The Sports Illustrated Book of Tennis*. Philadelphia: Lippincott, 1972

Tarshes, Barry, *Tennis & the Mind*. New York: Atheneum, 1977

VOLLEYBALL
Associations

U.S. Volleyball Association
422 Ninth Avenue
New York, New York 10001

Books

Peppler, Mary Jo, *Inside Volleyball for Women*. Chicago: Regnery, 1977

Robinson, Bonnie & Eds., *The Sports Illustrated Book of Volleyball*. Philadelphia: Lippincott, 1970

YOGA
Books

_____, *Yoga*. (Know the Game Series). New York: British Book Center, 1975

Brena, Stephen, *Yoga & Medicine*. New York: Penguin, 1973

Carr, Rachel, *Yoga for All Ages*. New York: Simon & Schuster, 1975

Diskin, Eve, *Yoga for Children*. New York: Warner Books, 1976

Hittleman, Richard, *Yoga for Personal Living*. New York: Warner Books, 1972

Hittleman, Richard, *Yoga for Physical Fitness*. New York: Warner Books, 1974

Nottidge, Pamela & Lamplugh, Diana, *Slimnastics*. New York: Penguin Books, 1973   ,

Ockford, William P. *Yoga: Gives Executives Time to Reduce Tension & Increase Productivity*. New York: Vantage Books.

Rawls, Eugene & Diskin, Eve, *Yoga for Beauty & Health: Look Younger & Be Relaxed*. New York: Warner Books, 1976

Spring, Clare & Goss, Madelaine, *Yoga for Today: The Way to Health & Beauty*. New York: Holt, Rinehart & Winston, 1959

Webb, Audrey T., *Slimming with Yoga*. New York: Essandess, 1970

Yisudian, Selvarajan & E. Haich, *Yoga & Health*. New York: Holt, Rinehart, & Winston, 1965

BEAUTY

Clark, Linda & Lee, Kay, *Beauty Questions & Answers*. New York: Pyramid Books, 1977

Glamour Magazine Editors, *Glamour Beauty Book*. New York: Simon & Schuster, 1972

Lawson, Donn & Conlon, Jean, *Beauty is No Big Deal*. New York: Bernard Geis, 1971

Seiffert, Dorothy, *Beauty for the Mature Woman*. New York: Hawthorn Books, 1977

Steinhart, Lawrence, M., *Beauty Through Health*. New York: Arbor House, 1974

Stillman, Irwin M., M.D. & Baker, Samm Sinclair, *Dr. Stillman's 14-Day Shape-up Program*. New York: Dell, 1974

Taylor, Eric, *Beautify Your Figure*. New York: Arc Books, 1972

Von Furstenberg, Diane, *Diane von Furstenberg's Book of Beauty*. New York: Simon & Schuster, 1977

STRESS

Benson, Herbert, *Relaxation Response*. New York: William Morrow, 1975.

Deming, Richard, Sleep, *Our Unknown Life*. New York: Thomas Nelson, 1972

Dunkell, Samuel, *Sleep Positions: The Night Language of the Body*. New York: William Morrow, 1976

Fink, David, *Release From Nervous Tension.* New York: Essandess, 1953

Fraser, Joan, *Relaxercises,* New York: Pinnacle Books, 1972

Janis, Irving L., *Stress & Frustration.* New York: Harcourt, Brace, Javonovich, 1971

Kastner, Jonathan & Kastner, Marianna., *Sleep: The Mysterious Third of Your Life.* New York: Harcourt, Brace, Jovanovich, 1968

Linde, Shirley, M., *Sleep Book.* New York: Harper & Row, 1974

Luce, Gay G. & Segal, Julius., *Sleep.* New York: Coward, McCann, Geoghegen, 1966

McQuade, Walter, & Aikman, Ann. *Stress.* New York: Bantam Books, 1975

Monat, Alan & Lazarus, Richard S., *Stress & Coping: An Anthology.* New York: Columbia University Press, 1977

Murray, Edward J., *Sleep, Dreams and Arousal.* Englewood Cliffs; Prentice-Hall, 1965

Oswald, Ian, *Sleep.* New York: Penguin Books, 1966

Selye, Hans, *Stress of Life.* New York: McGraw-Hill, 1976

Seyle, Hans, *Stress Without Distress,* New York: New American Library, 1975

SMOKING

Billingslea, Monro, *Smoking & How to Stop.* New York: Pageant-Poseiden, 1976

Ochsner, Alton, *Smoking: Your Choice Between Life & Death.* New York: Simon & Schuster, 1971

Royal College of Physicians of London, *Smoking & Health Now.* Philadelphia: Lippincott, 1971

ALCOHOLISM

Associations

Alcoholism Advisory, Consultation & Information Center
267 South Ocean Avenue
Freeport, New York
516–378–1491

Alcoholics Anonymous
Central Office
24 East 22nd Street
New York, New York 10016
212–GR3–6200

Alcoholics Anonymous General Services
468 Park Avenue South
New York, New York 10016
212–686–1100

Alcoholics Anonymous Grapevine
468 Park Avenue South
New York, New York 10016
212–686–1100

Alcoholics Anonymous World Services
468 Park Avenue South
New York, New York 10016
212–686–1100

Alcoholism Answering & Referral
730 Fifth Avenue
New York, New York 10022
212–765–0990

Alcoholism Center
300 Park Avenue South
New York, New York 10016
212–674–8850

Alcoholism Treatment
Smithers Center
Roosevelt Hospital
428 West 59th Street
New York, New York 10036
212–554–6721

Books

Block, Marvin H., *Alcohol & Alcoholism: Drinking & Dependence.* New York: Wadsworth, 1970

Coudert, Jo, *Alcohol in Your Life.* New York: Warner Books, 1974

Filstead, William J. Ed., *Alcohol & Alcohol Problems.* New York: Ballinger, 1976

Fort, Joel, *Alcohol: Our Biggest Drug Problem.* New York: McGraw-Hill, 1973

Kessell, Neil & Walton, Henry. *Alcoholism.* New York & London Penguin, 1966

Lyon Peter, & Fox, Ruth, *Alcoholism: It's Scope, Cause, & Treatment.* New York: Random House, 1955

Maxwell, Ruth., *Booze Battle: The Common Sense Approach That Works*. New York: Ballantine Books, 1977

Milt, Harry, *Alcoholism: Its Causes & Cure*. New York: Scribners, 1976

Pittman, David J., *Alcoholism*. New York: Harper & Row, 1967

Silverstein Alvin & Silverstein, Virginia B., *Alcoholism*. Philadelphia: Lippincott, 1976

Weiner, Jack B., *The Morning After*. New York: Dell, 1974

Williams, Roger A., *Alcoholism: The Nutritional Approach*. Austin: University of Texas Press, 1959

WORK & MONEY

Hennig, Margaret & Jardim, Anne, *The Managerial Woman*. New York: Anchor Press, 1977

Levinson, Harry, *Emotional Health in the World of Work*. New York: Harper & Row, 1964

Nelson, Paula, *The Joy of Money: The Guide to Women's Financial Freedom*. New York: Stein & Day, 1975

Porter, Sylvia, *Sylvia Porter's Money Book*. New York: Avon Books, 1976

PSYCHIATRIC HELP

Psychiatric Center of New York
139 East 37th Street
New York, New York 10017
212–683–7377

Psychiatric Research Foundation
130 East 77th Street
New York, New York 10021
212–249–1400

Psycho-Analytic Treatment Service
349 East 52nd Street
New York, New York 10022
212–838–4299

Psycho-Sexual Research Center
663 5th Avenue
New York, New York 10017
212–757–6454

Psychoanalytic Advisory & Referral Bureau
241 East 76th Street
New York, New York 10021
212–NA8–7100

PSYCHOLOGY, SEX, & HUMAN RELATIONS

Becker, Ernest, *The Denial of Death*. New York: The Free Press, 1974

Berne, Eric, *Games People Play*, Bantam

Comfort, Alex, *The Joy of Sex*. New York: A fireside Book, 1972

Comfort, Alex, *More Joy of Sex*. New York: A Fireside Book, 1974

DeRosis, Helen, M.D. and Victoria Y. Pellegrino, *The Book of Hope: How Women Can Overcome Depression*. New York: Bantam Books, 1977

Dyer, Wayne, *Your Erroneous Zones*, T.Y. Crowell, 1976, Avon, 1977

Fromm, Erich, *The Art of Loving*. New York: Harper & Row, 1956

Horney, Karen, M.D. *Neurosis & Human Growth*. New York: W. W. Norton & Company, 1950

Horney, Karen, M.D., *Feminine Psychology*. New York: W. W. Norton, 1943

Rubin, Theodore Isaac, M.D., *Understanding Your Man: A Woman's Guide*. New York: Ballentine, 1977

Sheehy, Gail, *Passages*. New York: Bantam Books, 1977

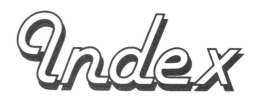

319